# Histological Typing of Urinary Bladder Tumours

W0227917

**Springer**
*Berlin*
*Heidelberg*
*New York*
*Barcelona*
*Hong Kong*
*London*
*Milan*
*Paris*
*Singapore*
*Tokyo*

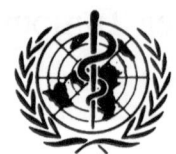 World Health Organization

The series *International Histological Classification of Tumours* consist of the following volumes. The early ones can be ordered through WHO, Distribution and Sales, Avenue Appia, CH-1211 Geneva 27.

2. Histological typing of breast tumours (1968, second edition 1981)
14. Histological and cytological typing of neoplastic diseases of haematopoietic and lymphoid tissues (1976)
22. Histological typing of prostate tumours (1980)
23. Histological typing of endocrine tumours (1980)

A coded compendium of the International Histological Classification of Tumours (1978)

*The following volumes have already appeared in a revised second edition with Springer-Verlag:*
Histological Typing of Thyroid Tumours. Hedinger/Williams/Sobin (1988)
Histological Typing of Intestinal Tumours. Jass/Sobin (1989)
Histological Typing of Oesophageal and Gastric Tumours. Watanabe/Jass/Sobin (1990)
Histological Typing of Tumours of the Gallbladder and Extrahepatic Bile Ducts. Albores-Saavedra/Henson/Sobin (1990)
Histological Typing of Tumours of the Upper Respiratory Tract and Ear. Shanmugaratnam/Sobin (1981)
Histological Typing of Salivary Gland Tumours. Seifert (1991)
Histological Typing of Odontogenic Tumours. Kramer/Pindborg/Shear (1992)
Histological Typing of Tumours of the Central Nervous System. Kleihues/Burger/Scheithauer (1993)
Histological Typing of Bone Tumours. Schajowicz (1993)
Histological Typing of Soft Tissue Tumours. Weiss (1994)
Histological Typing of Female Genital Tract Tumours. Scully et al. (1994)
Histological Typing of Tumours of the Liver. Ishak et al. (1994)
Histological Typing of Tumours of the Exocrine Pancreas. Klöppel/Solcia/Longnecker/Capella/Sobin (1996)
Histological Typing of Skin Tumours. Heenan/Elder/Sobin (1996)
Histological Typing of Cancer and Precancer of the Oral Mucosa. Pindborg/Reichart/Smith/van der Waal (1997)
Histological Typing of Kidney Tumours. Mostofi/Davis (1998)
Histological Typing of Testis Tumours. Mostofi/Sesterhenn (1998)
Histological Typing of Tumours of the Eye and Its Adnexa. Campbell (1998)
Histological Typing of Ovarian Tumours. Scully (1999)
Histological Typing of Lung and Pleural Tumours. Travis et al. (1999)
Histological Typing of Urinary Bladder Tumours. Mostofi et al. (1999)

# Histological Typing
# of Urinary Bladder Tumours

F. K. Mostofi, C. J. Davis and I. A. Sesterhenn

In Collaboration with L.H. Sobin
and Pathologists in 10 Countries

Second Edition

With 134 Colour Figures

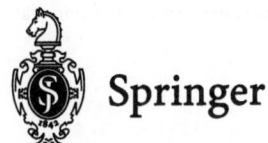 Springer

F. K. Mostofi, MD
Department of Genitourinary
Pathology,
Armed Forces Institute of Pathology,
Washington, DC 20306-6000, USA

I. A. Sesterhenn, MD
Department of Genitourinary
Pathology,
Armed Forces Institute of Pathology,
Washington, DC 20306-6000, USA

L. H. Sobin, MD
WHO Collaborating Center
for the International
Histological Classification of Tumours,
Armed Forces Institute of Pathology,
Washington, DC 20306-6000, USA

C. J. Davis, Jr., MD
Department of Genitourinary
Pathology,
Armed Forces Institute of Pathology,
Washington, DC 20306-6000, USA

First edition published by WHO in 1973 as No. 10 in the International Histological Classification of Tumours series

ISBN-13:978-3-540-64063-9

CIP data applied for

Die Deutsche Bibliothek – CIP-Einheitsaufnahme
International histological classification of tumours / World Health Organization. – Berlin; Heidelberg; New York; Barcelona; Hong Kong; London; Milan; Paris; Singapore; Tokyo: Springer
Mostofi, F. K.: Histological typing of urinary bladder tumours. – 2. ed. – 1999

Die Deutsche Bibliothek – CIP-Einheitsaufnahme
Mostofi, F. K.: Histological typing of urinary bladder tumours / F. K. Mostofi, C. J. Davis and I. A. Sesterhenn. In collab. with L. H. Sobin and pathologists in 10 countries. – 2. ed. – Berlin; Heidelberg; New York; Barcelona; Hong Kong; London; Milan; Paris; Singapore; Tokyo: Springer, 1999
  (International histological classification of tumours)
  ISBN-13:978-3-540-64063-9       e-ISBN-13: 978-3-642-59871-5
  DOI: 10.1007/978-3-642-59871-5

This work is subject to copyright. All rights are reserved, whether the whole or part of the material is concerned, specifically the rights of translation, reprinting, reuse of illustrations, recitation, broadcasting, reproduction on microfilm or in any other way, and storage in data banks. Duplication of this publication or parts thereof is permitted only under the provisions of the German Copyright Law of September 9, 1965, in its current version, and permission for use must always be obtained from Springer-Verlag. Violations are liable for prosecution under the German Copyright Law.

© Springer-Verlag Berlin Heidelberg 1999

The use of general descriptive names, registered names, trademarks, etc. in this publication does not imply, even in the absence of a specific statement, that such names are exempt from the relevant protective laws and regulations and therefore free for general use.

Product liability: The publishers cannot guarantee the accuracy of any information about the dosage and application contained in this book. In every individual case the user must check such information by consulting the relevant literature.

Typesetting: K+V Fotosatz, Beerfelden

SPIN 10665789   24/3135–5 4 3 2 1 0 – Printed on acid-free paper.

# Participants

*Algaba, F., Dr.*
Department of Pathology, Puigvert Foundation, Barcelona, Spain

*Andersson, L., Dr.*
WHO Collaborating Center for Urologic Tumours,
Department of Urology, Karolinska Hospital, Stockholm, Sweden

*Boccon-Gibod, L., Dr.*
Hospital Trousseau, Department of Pathology, Paris, France

*Busch, C., Dr.*
University Hospital, Department of Pathology, Tromso, Norway

*El-Bolkainy, M.N., Dr.*
National Cancer Institute of Cairo, Cairo, Egypt

*Davis Jr., C.J., Dr.*
Department of Genitourinary Pathology, Armed Forces Institute
of Pathology, Washington, DC

*Fukushima, S., Dr.*
Department of Pathology, Osaka City University Medical School,
Osaka, Japan

*Mostofi, F.K., Dr.*
Department of Genitourinary Pathology, Armed Forces Institute
of Pathology, Washington, DC

*Romanenko, A.M., Dr.*
Department of Pathology, Research Institute of Urology
and Nephrology, Kiev, Ukraine

*Sesterhenn, I. A., Dr.*
Department of Genitourinary Pathology, Armed Forces Institute
of Pathology, Washington, DC

*Suzigan, S., Dr.*
Department of Pathology, Larpac, Sao Paulo, Brazil

*Tribukait, B., Dr.*
Department of Medical Radiobiology, Karolinska Institute,
Stockholm, Sweden

*Webb, J. N., Dr.*
Western General Hospital, Department of Pathology,
Edinburgh, United Kingdom

*Zugan, H., Dr.*
Department of Pathology, Cancer Hospital, Beijing, China

# General Preface to the Series

Among the prerequisites for comparative studies of cancer are international agreement on histological criteria for the classification of cancer types and a standardized nomenclature. At present, pathologists use different terms for the same pathological entity, and, furthermore, the same term is sometimes applied to lesions of different types. An internationally agreed classification of tumours, acceptable alike to physicians, surgeons, radiologists, pathologists, and statisticians, would enable cancer workers in all parts of the world to compare their findings and would facilitate collaboration among them.

In a report published in 1952[1], a subcommittee of the WHO Expert Committee on Health Statistics discussed the general principles that should govern the statistical classification of tumours and agreed that, to ensure the necessary flexibility and ease in coding, three separate classifications were needed according to (1) anatomical site, (2) histological type, and (3) degree of malignancy. A classification according to anatomical site is available in the International Classification of Diseases[2].

In 1956, the WHO Executive Board passed a resolution[3] requesting the Director-General to explore the possibility that WHO might organize centres in various parts of the world and arrange for the collection of human tissues and their histological classification.

The main purpose of such centres would be to develop histological definitions of cancer types and to facilitate the wide adoption of a uniform nomenclature. This resolution was endorsed by the Tenth World Health Assembly in May 1957[4].

---

[1] WHO (1952) WHO Technical Report Series, no. 53. WHO, Geneva, p 45.
[2] WHO (1977) Manual of the international statistical classification of diseases, injuries, and causes of death, 1975 version. WHO, Geneva.
[3] WHO (1956) WHO Official Records, no. 68, p 14 (resolution EB 17.R40).
[4] WHO (1957) WHO Official Records, no. 79, p 467 (resolution WHA 10.18).

Since 1958, WHO has established a number of centres concerned with this subject. The result of this endeavor has been the International Histological Classification of Tumours, a multi-volume series whose first edition was published between 1967 and 1981. The present revised second edition aims to update the classifications, reflecting the progress in diagnoses and relevance of tumour types to clinical and epidemiologic features.

# Preface to the Histological Typing of Bladder Tumours – Second Edition

Although the normal histological anatomy of the urinary bladder is simple and most of the tumours affecting it are epithelial in origin, there has been a lack of agreement on standard pathological criteria for the diagnosis of carcinomas and their grading. Obviously, this lack of agreement has made it difficult to compare the results of therapy and epidemiological data. This statement holds true today in reference to some papillary tumours.

In 1973[1], in an attempt to provide uniformity, certain criteria were proposed for the diagnosis of carcinoma and, based on these criteria, three grades were described: Grade I for tumours with the least degree of cellular anaplasia, grade III for tumours with the most severe degree of anaplasia, and grade II for those in between.

At that time, the WHO Panel emphasised that the criteria for carcinoma were arbitrary and that most of the components of those criteria may be present in certain inflammatory, reactive or regenerative conditions. The criteria proposed in 1973 were to provide reproducibility for comparing the results of therapy and epidemiological studies. It was recognised that some tumours classified as carcinomas may in fact not behave as such. It was stated that "until a more sound scientific basis is found for distinguishing between benign and malignant tumours of the urinary bladder, these histological criteria are recommended".

Since 1973, it has become obvious that many tumours diagnosed as carcinomas – particularly grade I papillary carcinomas – did not progress to invasion and metastases and that a revision of the classification was necessary.

---

[1] Mostofi FK, Sobin LH, Torloni H (1973) Histological typing of urinary bladder tumours. Geneva, World Health Organization (International Histological Classification of Tumours, No. 10).

In anticipation of revising the classification, a set of questions was sent to 60 pathologists, urologists, cytologists, oncologists and basic scientists. Many of these individuals made very helpful, written comments and the following attended a conference at the Armed Forces Institute of Pathology in Washington, DC[2]:

Dr. F. Algaba, Puigvert Foundation, Barcelona, Spain

Dr. William C. Allsbrook, Medical College of Georgia, Augusta, GA

Dr. Mahul B. Amin, Henry Ford Hospital, Detroit, MI

Dr. Lennart Andersson, WHO Collaborating Center for Urologic Tumours, Department of Urology, Karolinska Hospital, Stockholm, Sweden

Dr. Robert W. Brinsko, Armed Forces Institute of Pathology, Washington, DC

Dr. Charles J. Davis, Jr., Armed Forces Institute of Pathology, Washington, DC

Dr. Jonathan I. Epstein, Johns Hopkins Hospital, Baltimore, MD

Dr. Yener S. Erozan, Johns Hopkins Hospital, Baltimore, MD

Dr. Shoji Fukushima, Osaka City University Medical School, Osaka, Japan

Dr. Donald Henson, National Cancer Institute, Bethesda, MD

Dr. Elia A. Ishak representing Dr. M. N. El-Bolkainy, Cairo, Egypt

Dr. Sonny L. Johansson, University of Nebraska Medical Center, Omaha, NE

Dr. Leopold G. Koss, Montefiore Medical Center, New York, NY

Dr. F. K. Mostofi, Armed Forces Institute of Pathology, Washington, DC

Dr. Howard S. Levin, The Cleveland Clinic, Cleveland, OH

Dr. S. Bruce Malkowicz, University of Pennsylvania, Philadelphia, PA

Dr. Edward M. Messing, University of Rochester Medical School, Rochester, NY

Dr. Victor E. Reuter, Memorial Sloan-Kettering Cancer Center, New York, NY

Dr. Alina M. Romanenko, Institute of Urology and Nephrology, Kiev, Ukraine

Dr. Kenneth W. Sapp, Armed Forces Institute of Pathology, Washington, DC

Dr. Isabell A. Sesterhenn, Armed Forces Institute of Pathology, Washington, DC

---

[2] Our appreciation to Schering Oncology/Biotech and to Anthra Pharmaceuticals for their generous contributions which made the Conference possible.

Dr. Raj Shekar, Armed Forces Institute of Pathology,
  Washington, DC
Dr. David Sidransky, Johns Hopkins Hospital, Baltimore, MD
Dr. Bernard Tribukait, Karolinska Institute, Stockholm, Sweden
Dr. John N. Webb, Western General Hospital, Edinburgh,
  United Kingdom
Dr. Wei Zhang, Armed Forces Institute of Pathology,
  Washington, DC.

On the first day, the participants reviewed the comments received from questionnaires and made recommendations for the WHO Panel.

On the second day, the WHO Scientific Panel members considered the recommendations of the group and endeavored to develop the revised WHO classification of urinary bladder tumours.

At the March 1998 meeting of the International Society of Urological Pathology in Boston organized by Dr. Jonathan Epstein, the classification of papillary and flat lesions was again discussed. In April 1998, a small meeting organized by Dr. Christer Busch was held in Norway, principally concerned with grading. These discussions contributed to the preliminary draft which was circulated to all the members of the WHO Panel listed on pp. V–VI. Their responses provided the basis for a new draft. After further communications among the participants, the present classification and explanatory notes were recommended for publication.

It will be appreciated, of course, that the classification reflects the present state of knowledge and that modifications are almost certain to be needed as experience accumulates. Although the present classification has been adopted by the members of the group, it necessarily represents a view from which some pathologists may wish to dissent. Nevertheless, it is hoped that, in the interests of international cooperation, all pathologists will use the classification as proposed. Criticism and suggestions for its improvement will be welcomed; these should be sent to the World Health Organization, 1211 Geneva 27, Switzerland.

The histological classification of bladder tumours, which appears on pp. 3–5, contains the morphology code numbers of the *International Classification of Diseases for Oncology* (ICD-O)[3] and the *Systematized Nomenclature of Medicine* (SNOMED)[4].

---

[3] World Health Organization (1990) *International classification of diseases for oncology* (ICD-O). Geneva.

[4] College of American Pathologists (1982) *Systematized nomenclature of medicine* (SNOMED). Chicago, IL.

The publications in the series, *International Histological Classification of Tumours* are not intended to serve as textbooks, but rather to promote the adoption of a uniform terminology that will facilitate communication among cancer workers. For this reason, literature references have intentionally been omitted and readers should refer to standard works for bibliographies.

# Contents

# Introduction

This classification is based primarily on the microscopic characteristics of tumours and, therefore, is concerned with morphologically identifiable cell types and histological patterns as seen with conventional light microscopy.

The term *tumour* is used synonymously with *neoplasm*. The phrase *tumour-like* is applied to lesions which clinically or morphologically resemble neoplasms, but do not behave biologically in a neoplastic manner. They are included in this classification because they give rise to problems in differential diagnosis and because of the unclear borderline between neoplasms and certain non-neoplastic lesions. Synonyms are listed only if they have been widely used, or if they are considered to be helpful for the understanding of the lesion.

Four segments have been revised: (1) The designation of epithelial cells. Traditionally, the epithelium of the urinary tract has been designated as transitional cell type. It is now generally recognized, however, that this is a special type of epithelium which more accurately should be designated as *urothelium* and the tumours as *urothelial carcinomas*. Since both terms are still widely used in common parlance and current literature, they are used interchangeably in this classification. (2) The creation of the category of papillary neoplasms of low malignant potential, which includes many of those previously classified as papillary grade I carcinoma in the 1973 scheme. (3) More detailed definition of grades, principally involving grade 1 tumours. (4) Distinguishing variants of urothelial carcinoma.

Although the emphasis of this classification is on histological typing, in the examination of bladder tumours, consideration should also be given to the degree of cellular anaplasia, extent of local spread, vascular and lymphatic invasion and the occurrence of metastasis. Several grading systems are in use and the one recommended utilizes three grades as described on p. 10.

In addition to histological assessment and growth pattern, the clinical and pathological classification of the extent of the tumour (staging) should be taken into account for the purposes of treatment and prognosis. Such a system of staging (TNM) has been developed by the International Union Against Cancer (see p. 29–31).

# Histological Classification
# of Urinary Bladder Tumours

## 1 Epithelial Tumours of the Bladder

*1.1* *Benign*
1.1.1 Urothelial (transitional cell) papilloma ......... 8120/0[1,2]
1.1.2 Urothelial (transitional cell) papilloma,
inverted type ............................ 8121/0
1.1.3 Squamous cell papilloma ................... 8052/0
1.1.4 Villous adenoma ......................... 8261/0

*1.2* *Papillary urothelial (transitional cell) neoplasm*
*of low malignant potential* .................. 8130/1

*1.3* *Malignant*
1.3.1 Urothelial (transitional cell) carcinoma ......... 8120/3
1.3.1.1 Papillary urothelial (transitional cell) carcinoma .. 8130/3
1.3.1.2 Infiltrating urothelial (transitional cell) carcinoma . 8120/3
1.3.1.3 Urothelial (transitional cell) carcinoma in situ .... 8120/2
1.3.1.4 Atypia/dysplasia ......................... 74000
1.3.1.5 Variants of urothelial (transitional cell) carcinoma
1.3.2 Squamous cell carcinoma .................. 8070/3
1.3.2.1 Verrucous carcinoma ...................... 8051/3
1.3.3 Adenocarcinoma .......................... 8140/3
1.3.4 Urachal carcinoma ....................... 8010/3
1.3.5 Clear cell adenocarcinoma .................. 8310/3
1.3.6 Small cell carcinoma ..................... 8041/3

---

[1] Morphology code of the International Classification of Diseases for Oncology (ICD-O) and the Systematized Nomenclature of Medicine (SNOMED).
[2] Behaviour is coded /0 for benign tumours, /1 for low or uncertain malignant potential or borderline malignancy, /2 for in situ lesions and /3 for malignant tumours.

# Definitions and Explanatory Notes

## 1      Epithelial Tumours of the Bladder

### 1.1      Benign

#### 1.1.1      Urothelial (transitional cell) papilloma (Figs. 1–4)

*A papillary tumour with a delicate fibrovascular stroma covered by urothelium indistinguishable from that of the normal bladder.*

    The lesion is characterised by discrete papillary fronds, with occasional branching in some cases, but without fusion. The stroma may show some oedema or inflammatory cells, the epithelium has no atypia and umbrella cells are prominent. Mitoses are rare and, if present, are basal in location and not abnormal. These lesions are rare, usually isolated, quite small and typically seen in patients under the age of 50.

    Rarely, papilloma may show extensive involvement of the mucosa. This is referred to as *diffuse papillomatosis.*

    *Synonyms:* exophytic papilloma, typical papilloma.

#### 1.1.2      Urothelial (transitional cell) papilloma, inverted type (Figs. 5, 6)

*A tumour with the characteristics of a transitional cell papilloma, but with an endophytic rather than an exophytic growth pattern.*

    Most of these are solitary, pedunculated or sessile and located in the bladder neck or trigone. The surface epithelium is smooth and histologically normal or slightly attenuated. Invaginations from the surface extend into the stroma to form a maze-like proliferation of anastomosing cords of transitional epithelium. The epithelium is normal with some spindling in the centre of the cords. Some will show squamous areas, and a few have glandular foci with goblet cells. Widely scattered neuroendocrine cells may be present. Mitoses are rare and usually absent. Some tumours show features of both papilloma and inverted papilloma. As defined above, they are without malignant potential but must be distinguished from low-grade carcinomas with a largely inverted growth pattern. These carcinomas lack the maze-like pattern, but exhibit, instead, lobules or plates of solid epithelial masses and usually surface papillations.

*Synonyms:* endophytic papilloma, inverted papilloma.

### 1.1.3    Squamous cell papilloma (Figs. 7, 8)

*A bland proliferation of squamous epithelium, usually having the cytological features of condyloma acuminatum identical to that seen in other sites.*

Condylomas are distinguished from other squamous papillomas by the presence of koilocytes and the demonstrable human papilloma virus (HPV) subtypes 6/11. Most of these are associated with urethral condylomas or follow long-standing cystostomy or indwelling catheter. Extensive acanthosis with deep, pushing margins typical of verrucous carcinoma is absent.

### 1.1.4    Villous adenoma (Fig. 9)

*A benign neoplasm in which papillary fronds covered by colonic-type glandular epithelium project into the lumen of the bladder or urachus.*

Tall, pseudostratified, colonic-type epithelium lines villous or tubulovillous fronds identical to villous adenomas of the large bowel. Nuclei are dark, elongated and basal in location. Prominent nucleoli or stromal invasion indicate malignant change. As with other forms of glandular metaplasia, there is a malignant potential.

## 1.2    Papillary urothelial (transitional cell) neoplasm of low malignant potential (Figs. 10–12)

*A papillary tumour of urothelium which resembles the typical papilloma, but which shows an increased cellular proliferation, exceeding six cell layers in thickness.*

Although the counting of cell layers is an approximation, these papillary tumours clearly exceed in thickness that of normal bladder epithelium. The pattern gives the impression of predominant order with minimal or no variation of architectural and nuclear features. The basal cells may show palisading and there is little or no alteration of cell polarity. Mitoses are infrequent and usually have a basal location. Umbrella cells are present and may or may not be prominent. As with papillomas and low-grade papillary carcinomas, these may show a prominent inverted growth pattern.

It is understood that this lesion does not progress to carcinoma in the overwhelming majority of cases. However, the patients have an increased risk of developing new papillary lesions which occasionally are of higher grade and capable of malignant progression. In the future it may become evident that these lesions are best designated as "urothelial papillomas of low malignant potential" rather than "papillary urothelial neoplasms of low malignant potential". Pathologists are encouraged to include the following when this diagnosis is made: "Patients with these tumours are at risk of developing new bladder tumours, usually of similar histology. However, occasionally the subsequent lesion is a carcinoma. Follow-up is warranted". This category includes many of the grade I papillary carcinomas of the 1973 WHO classification and grade I papillary urothelial tumours of European classifications.

*Synonym:* grade I transitional cell tumour.


## 1.3    Malignant

### 1.3.1    *Urothelial (transitional cell) carcinoma*

*Any malignant epithelial tumour of the bladder consisting entirely, partly or focally of anaplastic urothelium (transitional epithelium).*

The basic elements in the diagnosis of urothelial carcinoma are growth pattern, nuclear grade and tumour stage. The growth patterns include: *papillary, infiltrating, in situ and any combination thereof.* Papillary and infiltrating carcinomas are graded; in situ carcinomas are not graded.

To avoid confusion with the category discussed in Sect. 1.3.1.3 [urothelial (transitional cell) carcinoma in situ], it is strongly recommended that non-invasive papillary tumours not be referred to as "in situ".

1.3.1.1    Papillary urothelial (transitional cell) carcinoma
(Figs. 13–20)

*A neoplasm of urothelium on papillary fronds.*

Unlike the papillomas and papillary neoplasms of low malignant potential, these tumours show architectural disorder and nuclear atypia of variable degree which is graded on a scale of I–III, since the rate of progression differs significantly with each of the three grades. In tumours with variable histology, the tumour is graded according to the highest grade area, although it has not been established whether minute foci of high-grade tumour impact on the prognosis.

The epithelium of grade I urothelial carcinomas has an overall orderly appearance, but with easily recognisable variations of architectural and cytologic features. In contrast to the papillary urothelial neoplasms of low malignant potential, it is easy to recognise variations of nuclear polarity, size, shape and chromatin. Mitoses are infrequent, but may occur at any level of the epithelium, usually the basal third. Fronds should be evaluated where sectioned lengthwise through the core or when sectioned at right angles away from the base. Otherwise, there may be a misleading impression of increased cellularity and mitoses or loss of polarity.

Grade I papillary urothelial carcinomas as described herein correspond to some of those which were previously called grade I in the 1973 WHO classification. They also correspond to "low grade" urothelial carcinomas and to grade 2A carcinomas in many European centres.

Grade II tumours exhibit an intermediate degree of abnormality. They are distinguished from grade I by a predominately disordered architectural pattern, but with retention of some elements of organisation, e.g. polarity and nuclear uniformity. These elements are not seen in grade III. These features are unchanged from the previous WHO grade II carcinomas and correspond to grade 2B tumours in much of Europe. In the low grade–high grade scheme, they are included with the high grade lesions.

Grade III tumours present an overall impression of complete disorder or chaos with absence of polarity and, commonly, loss of superficial cells, marked variation of all nuclear parameters and, usually, numerous irregularly distributed mitoses. The grade III carcinomas are identical to the grade III lesions of the 1973 WHO classification, and correspond to the grade III tumours of European centres and to "high-grade" tumours of other centres.

With increasing grade epithelial thickness may be variable due to increasing loss of cellular cohesion.

In the classification and grading of papillary urothelial tumours, the most critical distinction is between the papillomas, papillary urothelial neoplasms of low malignant potential and grade I papillary carcinomas on the one hand and between grade II and grade III carcinomas on the other.

### 1.3.1.2    Infiltrating urothelial (transitional cell) carcinoma (Figs. 21–26)

*A urothelial tumour that invades beyond the basement membrane.*

As with the papillary tumours these are graded on a I–III scale, depending upon the degree of nuclear anaplasia. The most anaplastic areas determine the tumour grade. Again, some centres divide these lesions into "low-grade" and "high-grade" categories.

In addition to grade, the manner of stromal invasion should be reported since those tumours which exhibit broad-front or pushing margins are less aggressive than those with tentacular growth. Three other patterns of invasive growth, described below as variants, should be included in the diagnosis for the purpose of future study and comparison: micropapillary, microcystic and nested.

Pathological staging should be done on all bladder specimens. The TNM system is recommended and the report should include the specific anatomic information upon which the staging was based in order to avoid any misunderstanding.

The distinction between lamina propria invasion and tangential sections through surface epithelium or von Brunn nests can be difficult, but is important. With non-invasive lesions, the basement membrane preserves a smooth, regular contour which differs from the irregular contours of invasive aggregates. Thin-walled vessels often line basement membranes of non-invasive nests. With invasive lesions, the character of the adjacent stroma often differs from that seen in other areas, e.g. fibrosis, sclerosis and retraction artefacts. The last are frequently mistaken for lymphatic or vascular invasion. When the space contains no blood, lymphocytes or obvious endothelial cell lining, this is likely to represent shrinkage artefact.

Lamina propria invasion should be described as focal or extensive, but the term "superficial bladder cancer" should not be used since it lumps together two biologically different lesions (pTa and pT1). The thin, usually discontinuous fascicles of the muscularis mucosae should not be confused with the thick fascicles of the muscularis propria. The former are found approximately in the mid lamina propria, parallel to the surface and often associated with prominent vessels. The term "muscle invasion" is inadequate histologically because it does not distinguish between muscularis mucosae and muscularis propria or between superficial and deep muscle invasion.

Pathology reports should mention whether muscularis propria is present or absent, in order to inform the urologist as to the depth of the biopsy.

On transurethral resections, one should not attempt to subclassify muscularis propria invasion. Since adipose tissue can be seen in lamina propria and muscularis propria, deep muscle invasion (pT2b) can be diagnosed with certainty only on total or partial cystectomy specimens.

### 1.3.1.3    Urothelial (transitional cell) carcinoma in situ (Figs. 27–36)

*A non-papillary, i.e. flat, lesion in which the surface epithelium contains cells that are cytologically malignant.*

The neoplastic change may or may not involve the entire thickness of the epithelial layer. It may be present in only the surface layer or only the basal layer, or it may be pagetoid, with individual or groups of neoplastic cells scattered amidst apparently normal urothelial cells. It may involve von Brunn nests or cystitis cystica. The fragile epithelium may be severely damaged either spontaneously or by biopsy forceps so that only a few residual cancer cells remain on the surface ("clinging carcinoma in situ"). This definition includes lesions that were previously classified as severe dysplasia and some cases of moderate dysplasia.

*Synonym:* high-grade intraurothelial neoplasia.

### 1.3.1.4    Atypia/dysplasia (Figs. 37, 38)

Either of these terms apply to urothelium which is not normal, but the cytologic and architectural alterations are insufficient to warrant a diagnosis of carcinoma in situ.

*Synonym:* low-grade intraurothelial neoplasia.

### 1.3.1.5    Variants of urothelial (transitional cell) carcinoma

The potentiality of malignant urothelium is reflected in the wide range of variant morphologies of invasive lesions. Some of these are common, others are rare; some represent variations of invasive growth patterns, others of cellular morphology. For purposes of future study and comparison of different therapeutic modalities, it is recommended that these variants be incorporated into the diagnosis.

*Urothelial (transitional cell) carcinoma with squamous and/or glandular metaplasia* (Figs. 39–42) is the designation applied to those transitional cell carcinomas with foci or extensive areas of malignant squamous and/or glandular epithelium. This is a common variant that includes, in addition to areas resembling squamous cell carcinoma or adenocarcinoma (or both), an element of urothelial carcinoma. The latter may be confined to the surface epithelium. For these lesions, the recommended diagnosis is: "urothelial (or transitional cell) carcinoma (grade), with glandular (or squamous) metaplasia, (level of invasion)".

*Spindle cell carcinoma* (Figs. 43–45) refers to those transitional (or squamous) carcinomas that contain a predominance of spindle cells. These tumours proliferate as fascicles or storiform lesions which mimic various sarcomas or myofibroblastic tumours. In most cases, areas of differentiated carcinoma will be evident, particularly when highlighted with epithelial markers (cytokeratin or epithelial membrane antigen). Wide sampling may be required to identify such areas, as well as carcinoma in situ which is usually present.

*Synonym:* sarcomatoid carcinoma.

*Urothelial carcinoma with lymphocytic infiltrate* (Figs. 46–48) is the diagnosis for some invasive carcinomas that are associated with an intense infiltration of lymphocytes. These may be confused with lymphoproliferative lesions. Various degrees of epithelial differentiation may be seen, but epithelial markers are invariably positive. Poorly differentiated lesions may be obscured by lymphocytes or occasionally plasma cells, neutrophils or eosinophils. This has been designated "*lymphoepithelioma-like carcinoma*".

*Osteoclastic variant* (Fig. 49) refers to those urothelial carcinomas that are associated with numerous cells within the stroma that are indistinguishable from osteoclasts. These tumours are classified and graded, however, without regard to the giant cells, which are likely a reaction to the tumour rather than a determinant of its behaviour.

Other types of stromal reaction to bladder neoplasia include bizarre, multinucleated or otherwise atypical mesenchymal stromal cells, similar to those associated with radiation cystitis (see Sect. 7.11). Cytologically benign deposits of bone or cartilage rarely are found in the stroma adjacent to tumours.

*Urothelial carcinoma, clear cell variant* (Figs. 50, 51) includes urothelial carcinomas that exhibit extensive areas of optically clear, glycogen-rich cytoplasm. Typical papillary or in situ lesions are generally present and the tubular, microcystic and hobnail features of clear cell adenocarcinoma (see Sect. 1.3.5) are absent.

*Urothelial carcinoma with ectopic placental glycoprotein production* (Figs. 52–55) applies to those urothelial carcinomas which produce trophoblastic hormones, usually beta-human chorionic gonadotropin. These are usually high-grade lesions with bizarre mononuclear or multinuclear cells. Rarely, the cells have a resemblance to syncytiotrophoblasts, but, unlike choriocarcinoma, immunoreactivity is not confined to the giant cells.

*Plasmacytoid variant* (Figs. 56, 57) refers to those invasive tumours in which the cells present a plasmacytoid appearance. Epithelial markers are invariably positive and cytoplasmic mucin can be demonstrated in most cases.

Typical signet-ring cells may also be present. When urothelial elements are present, such as in situ carcinoma, the recommended diagnosis is: "Transitional cell (or urothelial) carcinoma, poorly differentiated plasmacytoid variant". In pure form, i.e. without a transitional cell component, these should be coded as "adenocarcinoma, poorly differentiated, plasmacytoid variant".

*Lipid cell variant* (Figs. 58, 59) is a urothelial carcinoma which exhibits transition to a cell type resembling signet-ring lipoblasts. These cells may comprise the bulk of the tumour, but typical features of urothelial carcinoma are generally present. This is an ill-defined and uncommon variant which has been considered in several instances as carcinoma with liposarcoma. It remains to be established whether this should be classified as carcinosarcoma.

*Micropapillary variant* (Figs. 60–62) refers to a morphologic growth pattern assumed by many invasive carcinomas. Small aggregates of tumour cells with indistinct stromal cores are associated with retraction artefacts that mimic vascular invasion. These are high-grade tumours, usually occurring with more typical areas of transitional cell carcinoma.

*Nested variant* (Figs. 63, 64) is a urothelial carcinoma that infiltrates as small, rounded cell aggregates which resemble nests of von Brunn. These differ from benign nests, however, in that they show more variation in size and contour and have mild nuclear atypia. At deeper levels, atypia usually increases and cell aggregates are more pleomorphic in size and shape.

In the *microcystic variant* (Figs. 65–67) the invasive element of urothelial carcinoma is composed of rounded, oval or elongated cysts 1–2 mm in size. These are generally associated with typical areas of urothelial carcinoma.

### 1.3.2     Squamous cell carcinoma (Figs. 68, 69)

*A malignant tumour consisting entirely of squamous cells without urothelial or glandular elements.*

Microscopically, most of these are moderately or well-differentiated tumours, with clearly evident keratinisation and intercellular bridges. Most invade deeply into the muscularis propria. Squamous metaplasia is generally present in the bladder epithelium adjacent to the tumour. This usually occurs in a setting of chronic irritation such as stones, indwelling catheters, infection or diverticula, conditions conducive to the development of keratinising squamous metaplasia. Squamous cell carcinoma is the most frequent carcinoma in schistosomiasis.

#### 1.3.2.1     Verrucous carcinoma (Fig. 70)

*An exophytic well-differentiated squamous cell carcinoma with minimal nuclear atypia and with papillomatosis and rounded acanthotic extensions pushing deeply into the stroma without true stromal invasion.*

This variant of squamous cell carcinoma is rare except where schistosomiasis is endemic. Some have condylomatous features with demonstrable HPV 6/11.

### 1.3.3     Adenocarcinoma (Figs. 71–74)

*A malignant glandular neoplasm arising from bladder epithelium which contains no urothelial or squamous elements and is not of urachal origin.*

Most of these are similar to adenocarcinomas of the large intestine and may be glandular, mucinous (colloid) or of signet-ring cell-type. Bladder adenocarcinomas arise from glandular metaplasia of urothelium and, in many cases, areas of cystitis glandularis or intestinal metaplasia will be evident in or adjacent to the tumour. Some

form of chronic irritation is often in the history, including schistosomiasis, although most of those are squamous cell tumours. Adenocarcinoma is the common tumour in extrophy.

### 1.3.4 Urachal carcinoma (Figs. 75, 76)

*A malignant epithelial tumour, usually glandular, in the dome or ad-*
*jacent anterior bladder wall with an epicentre in the muscularis pro-*
*pria or deeper, arising from remnants of the urachal tract.*

The majority of these are of the mucinous (colloid) type with columnar or signet-ring cells floating within lakes of mucin which are
located chiefly in the muscularis propria rather than the lamina propria. Less commonly, the tumour may be of the moderately or well-
differentiated enteric type or the linitis plastica signet-ring cell-type.
Some tumours occur in the urachal tract above the bladder and may
present at the umbilicus. Urothelial and squamous cell carcinomas in
the dome usually prove to be of bladder origin, although these very
rarely will be urachal if other criteria are met. Since special stains
and immunohistochemistry do not distinguish between urachal, bladder and metastatic adenocarcinomas, it should be established that the
tumour is in the dome or adjacent anterior bladder wall, chiefly in the
muscularis propria or deeper and that the adjacent bladder mucosa is
non-neoplastic. Glandular or intestinal metaplasia of the bladder
would suggest a bladder primary. Colonic carcinoma involving the
bladder must be specifically ruled out.

### 1.3.5 Clear cell adenocarcinoma (Figs. 77–79)

*An adenocarcinoma with a tubular growth pattern and clear cell or*
*hobnail cytological features.*

Usually seen in the urethra, these rarely are found in the bladder.
Microscopically, the tumour forms tubules rather than glands and
may also form microcysts and papillations. The cells are generally
clear or partially clear in most areas and often have a hobnail appearance. The cells have abundant glycogen and, usually, focal cytoplasmic and luminal mucin. They differ from nephrogenic adenomas by
showing nuclear stratification, cellular anaplasia and mitoses and by
the absence of basement membranes. Either lesion, however, may ex-
tend into the muscularis propria.

Some urothelial carcinomas have a clear cell morphology with glycogen and mucin, but they are not tubular (see Sect. 1.3.1.5, urothelial carcinoma, clear cell variant). Metastatic renal cell carcinomas are distinguishable by their endocrine-like vascularity and absence of mucin. Metastatic clear cell carcinoma of the female genital tract must be excluded.

*Synonyms:* mesonephric carcinoma, tubular carcinoma.

### 1.3.6    Small cell carcinoma (Fig. 80)

This malignant tumour is identical to that occurring in the lung. Urothelial carcinoma in situ can be demonstrated in most cases and there are frequently areas of squamous, glandular or other variants of urothelial tumours. Lacking these elements, metastatic disease must be considered, as well as extension from a primary prostatic small cell carcinoma.

*Synonym:* small cell neuroendocrine carcinoma.

### 1.3.7    Undifferentiated carcinoma (Fig. 81)

*A malignant epithelial tumour that is too poorly differentiated to be placed in any of the other categories of carcinoma.*

## 2    Non-epithelial Tumours (Figs. 82–90)

Soft tissue tumours of the bladder are classified according to the terminology and diagnostic criteria set forth in the *World Health Organization Histological Typing of Soft Tissue Tumours**.

*Leiomyomas* and *haemangiomas* are the most common benign soft tissue tumours of the bladder and do not differ from those occurring elsewhere. *Granular cell tumours and neurofibromas* are rare, the latter occurring usually in patients with von Recklinghausen disease.

*Rhabdomyosarcoma* is the common sarcoma of childhood; it usually presents as polypoid masses in the trigone–bladder neck area (sarcoma botryoides) and is typically of the embryonal type. There is

---

* Weiss SW (1994) World Health Organization. Histological Typing of Soft Tissue Tumours. Second Edition. Springer-Verlag, Heidelberg.

an invasive proliferation of undifferentiated cells in a myxoid stroma with a subepithelial zone of concentrated tumour cells (the cambium layer). Diagnostic strap cells with cross striations may not be found, particularly in biopsies, but a diagnosis can generally be established by immunohistochemistry.

*Leiomyosarcoma* is the common sarcoma of adults and does not differ from those occurring elsewhere. The differential diagnosis of leiomyosarcoma includes spindle cell (sarcomatoid) carcinoma and myofibroblastic proliferations, since these three constitute the great majority of spindle cell bladder lesions. Wide sampling may be needed to find in situ or differentiated foci of carcinoma in the spindle cell carcinoma. Myofibroblastic lesions are discussed in Sect. 7.5. Malignant fibrous histiocytoma, haemangiopericytoma, osteosarcoma, angiosarcoma, liposarcoma and rhabdoid tumours are rare.

# 3    Miscellaneous Tumours

## 3.1    Paraganglioma (Figs. 91–93)

Paragangliomas of the bladder are identical to those occurring elsewhere, consisting of discrete aggregates of cells ("zellballen") separated by a network of vascular channels.

The cells have eosinophilic or darker cytoplasm and in some cases have a striking resemblance to those of the adrenal medulla. Some nuclear variation may be present but mitoses are rare and usually absent. These are intramural lesions and, at the periphery, in proximity to the mucosa, the cells may have a smaller, neuroblastoma-like appearance. Distinction from invasive transitional cell carcinomas can be facilitated by the use of immunohistochemistry. Some bladder paragangliomas exist as small, compact neoplasms, while others are widely dispersed through the muscularis propria. Recognition of the malignant ones (12%–15%) generally requires the demonstration of nodal metastasis or extravesical extension.

*Synonym:* phaeochromocytoma.

## 3.2    Haematopoietic and lymphoid neoplasms (Fig. 94)

Lymphomas and plasmacytomas in the bladder do not differ from those occurring elsewhere. The majority are part of a systemic disease; primary lymphoma or plasmacytoma of bladder is uncommon.

Most of the lymphomas are of diffuse large cell or small lymphocytic types and are of B-cell origin. Follicular, mantle cell and plasmacytoid types are much less common. Except at autopsy, Hodgkin disease and leukemic infiltrates are rare.

## 3.3    Carcinosarcoma (Figs. 95–97)

*A neoplasm containing malignant epithelial and malignant heterologous mesenchymal elements.*

These tumours contain transitional, squamous or glandular tissue as the carcinomatous element and a mesenchymal element which can be identified specifically as sarcoma. Most commonly, the sarcoma will be osteosarcoma, chondrosarcoma, rhabdomyosarcoma or some combination of these. (Some centres include spindle cell carcinomas in this category.)

*Synonym:* malignant mixed mesodermal tumour.

## 3.4    Malignant melanoma (Figs. 98, 99)

Primary melanomas of bladder are rare and do not differ histologically, biologically or by immunohistochemistry from those seen elsewhere.

Many patients dying of malignant melanoma have bladder metastasis and when considering a diagnosis of primary vesicle melanoma, certain criteria should be met: no history of prior cutaneous, ophthalmic or other melanoma should be evident; examination of all skin surfaces should be negative and the metastatic pattern should be consistent with a bladder primary. Atypical melanocytes in the bladder epithelium will support a diagnosis of primary melanoma.

# 4    Metastatic Tumours and Secondary Extensions
## (Fig. 100)

Primary extravesical tumours are occasionally manifested initially in the bladder. The primary cancers that most frequently affect the bladder are those arising in the prostate, cervix and colon, spreading to the bladder by direct extension.

# 5    Unclassified Tumours

These are primary benign or malignant tumours that cannot with certainty be placed into any of the categories described above.

# 6    Epithelial Abnormalities

## 6.1    Hyperplasia

Hyperplasia describes a group of lesions lined by increased numbers of cytologically normal urothelial cells. Two types, described in the following two sections, are recognized.

### 6.1.1    Flat urothelial (transitional cell) hyperplasia (Fig. 101)

*The epithelium is increased in thickness and evidence of maturation from base to surface is generally evident.* This is not known to have unfavourable prognostic significance.

### 6.1.2    Papillary urothelial (transitional cell) hyperplasia
(Fig. 102)

*A lesion characterised by slight "tenting", undulating, micropapillary or pseudopapillary growth lined by urothelium lacking atypia.*
    Thickness of the epithelium is variable. This lesion often has a small, dilated capillary at its base, but it lacks a well-developed fibrovascular core. Its possible relationship to carcinoma is unknown, but some data suggest that it may represent a precursor of low-grade papillary urothelial neoplasia.

## 6.2    Reactive atypia (Figs. 103, 104)

This comprises mild epithelial abnormalities such as variations in nuclear size and staining and increased thickness of epithelium deemed to be non-neoplastic. These must be interpreted in the context of other findings. The cells are often larger than normal, with more abundant cytoplasm and there may be nucleoli. These features impart a squamoid appearance to reactive atypia. Chronic inflammation, lithiasis, recent instrumentation, catheters, or underlying tumours will produce cellular alterations which fall short of the generally accepted criteria for cytological malignancy. Some cases occur without apparent cause.

### 6.3    Atypia of uncertain significance (Figs. 105, 106)

In some cases it is difficult to distinguish between neoplastic and reactive atypia.

There may be a greater degree of pleomorphism and/or hyperchromasia disproportionate to the degree of inflammation, such that early neoplasia cannot be ruled out with certainty. Follow-up is indicated for these patients.

### 6.4    Von Brunn nests (Fig. 107)

*Compact, rounded aggregates of urothelial (transitional) cells in the lamina propria, with or without connection to the surface epithelium.*

These structures are present in most bladders, more commonly in the trigone. When numerous, they may produce a sessile or polypoid lesion and be mistaken cytoscopically for a tumour. Microscopically they can exhibit the same metaplastic and neoplastic processes which affect the adjacent surface epithelium. Tumour-like aggregates of von Brunn nests have some similarities to the inverted papilloma, but lack the branching or anastomosing feature of the latter.

Nests that show size variation and dispersion in the lamina propria may mimic the nested variant of urothelial carcinoma (see Sect. 1.3.1.5).

### 6.5    Cystitis cystica (Fig. 108)

*Aggregates of urothelial (transitional) cells located in the lamina propria and having central lumina.*

Evolving from von Brunn nests, cystitis cystica has a central lumen lined by flattened urothelial cells or eosinophilic columnar cells. As with von Brunn nests, florid proliferations may mimic neoplasia.

### 6.6    Glandular metaplasia (Figs. 109–111)

*Mucus-containing epithelial cells of colonic type lining the surface of the bladder lumen or forming glands in the lamina propria.*

Epithelial cells of colonic type with goblet cells (and rarely Paneth, argentaffin or argyrophil cells) constitute glandular metaplasia. This is seen most often in association with cystitis cystica and is designated *cystitis glandularis*. It may also involve surface epithelium. The latter has been designated *intestinal metaplasia* and it may have a striking resemblance to intestinal mucosa. Florid examples of glandular metaplasia are often associated with lakes of mucin in the adjacent stroma. Cellular atypia, manifested by nuclear pleomorphism and prominent nucleoli, is indicative of malignant change. Extensive metaplasia is a significant risk factor for adenocarcinoma.

### 6.7    Nephrogenic adenoma (Figs. 112–114)

*A non-neoplastic epithelial lesion consisting of cuboidal cells lining the bladder lumen or tubules within the lamina propria.*

Cuboidal metaplasia of urothelium followed by proliferation into the lamina propria of tubules with a similarity to renal tubules constitutes the nephrogenic adenoma. The bladder lumen may have a papillary or polypoid contour, lined by small, uniform cuboidal cells and the stromal element may include microcysts lined by hobnail cells and also mucin-containing cells resembling signet-ring cells. The latter, however, as well as the tubular lesions, often have prominent basement membranes, distinguishing these lesions from signet-ring cell carcinomas. The adjacent stroma is usually inflammatory with numerous lymphocytes and plasma cells. This type of metaplasia typically follows long-standing irritation such as stones or trauma, but most occur at the site of a prior surgical procedure. A malignant potential has not been demonstrated.

*Synonym:* adenomatous metaplasia.

### 6.8    Squamous metaplasia (Fig. 115)

*The replacement of transitional epithelium by squamous epithelium, either keratinizing or non-keratinizing.*

Squamous epithelium similar to that of vaginal mucosa is normally found in the trigone and bladder neck of most women in the reproductive age range and should not be regarded as metaplasia. Metaplastic squamous epithelium is commonly seen in a setting of chronic irritation such as stones, diverticuli, non-functioning bladders or schistosomiasis. Keratinizing squamous metaplasia (leukoplakia) constitutes a significant risk factor for the development of carcinoma, and most squamous cell carcinomas of the bladder arise from areas of keratinizing squamous metaplasia.

## 6.9    Treatment effects (Figs. 116–119)

Topical and certain systemic chemotherapeutic agents produce epithelial changes that can be mistaken for carcinoma. Thiotepa and Mitomycin C produce atypical changes in the superficial umbrella cells. These become large, vacuolated and often multinucleated with small nucleoli. Cellular changes induced by these agents are not specific and may be caused by chronic irritation.

Cyclophosphamide characteristically produces large, degenerated cells with high nuclear-cytoplasmic ratios and smudged nuclear chromatin. These features will generally be regarded as suspicious for in situ carcinoma, requiring close follow-up, particularly since this agent may be associated with bladder carcinoma. Haemorrhagic cystitis and bladder fibrosis are other complications.

Bacillus Calmette-Guérin (BCG) may produce denudation of epithelium and ulceration, but significant epithelial changes are not present other than reactive atypia. Small, superficial non-caseating granulomas and chronic inflammation comprise the usual findings with BCG therapy.

Radiation therapy results in cellular enlargement, multinucleation and vacuolisation, but nuclear-cytoplasmic ratios remain low. Enlarged nuclei may have large nucleoli, but degenerative nuclear features are usually present. In chronic cases, the hyperplastic and stromal changes noted in Sect. 7.11 will be evident.

## 7    Tumour-like Lesions

## 7.1    Papillary and polypoid cystitis (Figs. 120, 121)

*Exophytic lesions of the mucosa, resulting from inflammation or oedema, which resemble papillary neoplasms.*

With inflammation or oedema of the lamina propria, the mucosal surface assumes a papillary or polypoid contour, but the morphology of true neoplastic fronds is absent. Papillary neoplasms are composed of narrow fibrovascular cores lined by epithelium, whereas the polypoid lesions generally have a broad-based or club-shaped appearance due to oedema or other inflammatory changes. In difficult cases, the clinical setting should be taken into consideration. Indwelling catheters and fistulae are particularly likely to show these changes.

## 7.2     Follicular cystitis (Fig. 122)

*The occurrence of lymphoid follicles, usually with germinal centers in the lamina propria and infrequently in the muscularis propria.*

The tumour-like nature of follicular cystitis is due largely to the presence of small white or pink nodules, often on an erythematous mucosal surface, when viewed cystoscopically. Microscopically, the adjacent epithelium may exhibit reactive atypia, but a significant number of bladder carcinomas have been associated with follicular cystitis. Rare examples of follicular lymphoma can be distinguished from benign follicles using the same criteria applied elsewhere.

## 7.3     Malakoplakia (Fig. 123)

*Aggregates of eosinophilic macrophages with characteristic cytoplasmic inclusions within the superficial lamina propria.*

The lesions, usually multiple, occur as nodules or plaques and frequently resemble tumours cystoscopically. Lymphocytes and plasma cells are usually present but most of the cells are large, granular and eosinophilic macrophages. A variable number of these von Hansemann histiocytes contain the diagnostic Michaelis-Gutmann inclusions: spherical 5–8-μm bodies, with a targetoid or bull's eye appearance that may be highlighted with stains for iron, calcium or the periodic acid–Schiff reaction.

## 7.4     Amyloidosis (Fig. 124)

*The deposition of amyloid within the lamina propria and superficial zone of the muscularis propria.*

Presenting as gross hematuria, this shows ulcerated, nodular or polypoid lesions which are usually cystoscopically indistinguishable from carcinoma. Microscopically, masses of amyloid occupy the lamina propria, the adjacent muscle and, occasionally, blood vessels. There may be an associated giant cell reaction, and the amyloid material usually presents a fragmented or "shattered" appearance which distinguishes it from chronic oedema. Most cases occur as solitary lesions and as primary amyloidosis. Secondary amyloidosis is rare.

## 7.5    Myofibroblastic proliferations

### 7.5.1    *Myofibroblastic tumour* (Fig. 125)

*A tumour-like proliferation of myofibroblasts.*

Microscopically, most cases show an oedematous or myxoid stroma separating spindled or stellate eosinophilic cells in a manner reminiscent of a "tissue culture" appearance. In areas with a more compact growth, fascicles may be formed, but unlike myxoid leiomyosarcoma, a delicate vascular network and some inflammatory cells are often present. Mitoses are frequent but not abnormal. Deep penetration through the muscularis propria may occur and lesions may recur, but progression beyond the bladder has not been seen. Immunohistochemical reactivity of myofibroblasts and absence of in situ carcinoma distinguish these from spindled carcinomas. Frequent cytokeratin reactivity and the "tissue culture" growth pattern are helpful in distinguishing these from leiomyosarcoma. Their nature is unclear.

*Synonym:* inflammatory pseudotumour.

### 7.5.2    *Postoperative spindle cell nodule* (Fig. 126)

*A proliferation of myofibroblasts at the site of a prior surgical procedure.*

An exuberant, friable mass of tissue develops at the surgical site usually within 1–3 months after the event. The microscopic picture does not differ significantly from that of the inflammatory pseudotumour described in Sect. 7.5.1, although cellular growth is generally more compact and a merging with obvious granulation tissue is often present. A history of recent surgery is most helpful in excluding malignancy.

## 7.6    Fibrous (fibroepithelial) polyp (Fig. 127)

*A polypoid lesion composed of a fibrovascular stroma and lined by urothelial (transitional) epithelium.*

These are usually solitary and resemble fibroepithelial polyps seen elsewhere. The epithelium may be ulcerated or show squamous metaplasia, but it is not usually hyperplastic. The stroma is typically sparsely cellular, oedematous and often congested with some inflammatory cells. Scattered smooth muscle cells may be present. Bizarre stellate stromal cells may be seen, rarely.

## 7.7    Endometriosis (Figs. 128, 129)

This consists of endometrial glands and stroma in the bladder identical to endometriosis seen elsewhere. Thickening of the bladder wall, a palpable supra-pubic mass or cystic, haemorrhagic or oedematous mucosal changes can raise the possibility of bladder neoplasia. Microscopically, some of the glands may lack a stromal element, and some foci may show evidence of recent or remote haemorrhage. The lamina propria, muscularis propria or serosa may be involved. A similar distribution of glands may show the features of endocervix (*endocervicosis*). These glands occur as rounded or stellate-shaped structures scattered randomly in the bladder wall. The epithelium consists of a row of cuboidal or columnar cells with pale, mucin-positive cytoplasm. Ciliated cells are also present in some of these glands. Least commonly, glandular inclusions may assume a tubal-type morphology (*endosalpingiosis*).

## 7.8    Hamartoma

*A lesion similar to the fibroepithelial polyp, but containing nodular aggregates of von Brunn nests or cystitis cystica within a fibrous or muscular stroma.*

Von Brunn nests, cystitis cystica and occasionally glandular metaplasia or renal-like tubules occupy a cellular fibrous or myomatous stroma. Large polyps occurring in children suggest this diagnosis, although a clear distinction from a polypoid, proliferative cystitis may not be possible or essential.

## 7.9    Cysts (Fig. 130)

Most bladder cysts are of urachal origin, occurring in the anterior wall or dome. Urachal cysts arise from persistent remnants of the urachal tract and will be lined by transitional epithelium or flattened atrophic cells. Colonic metaplasia is often present. The lesion may be multilocular and, unless complicated by abscess or neoplasia, is typically asymptomatic.

Rare cloacal cysts are found in the posterior bladder wall and mullerian cysts occur in men between the bladder and rectum. Trigonal cysts contain normal urothelium and are also regarded as developmental anomalies. Some may be mullerian.

## 7.10    Schistosomiasis (Fig. 131)

Inflammatory polyps and ulcerations may be associated with mucosal deposition of schistosomal eggs. Prior to the development of neoplasia, vesical schistosomiasis produces tumour-like inflammatory lesions. Deposition of eggs in the lamina propria and muscularis propria is associated with an acute inflammatory reaction (neutrophils and eosinophils), followed by the formation of discrete granulomas with ulceration or polypoid masses involving the mucosa. Ova eventually become calcified and the bladder wall fibrotic. Imaging studies will detect calcific deposits and variable filling defects.

## 7.11    Radiation cystitis (Figs. 132–134)

*A reactive, tumour-like epithelial proliferation associated with haemorrhage, fibrin deposits, fibrinoid vascular changes and multinucleated stromal cells due to ionising radiation.*

The tumour-like phase of radiation cystitis usually occurs months or years following the radiation. Nodules of squamoid epithelium push into the lamina propria without evidence of true infiltrative growth. The adjacent tissue is haemorrhagic with deposits of fibrin and, deeper within the stroma, mesenchymal cells are often large and multinucleated ("giant cell cystitis"). Extensive scarring of the bladder wall is common.

# TNM Classification of Tumours of the Urinary Bladder[1]

## Rules for Classification

The classification applies only to carcinomas. Papilloma is excluded. There should be histological or cytological confirmation of the disease.

The following are the procedures for assessing T, N and M categories:

| | |
|---|---|
| *T categories* | Physical examination, imaging and endoscopy |
| *N categories* | Physical examination and imaging |
| *M categories* | Physical examination and imaging |

## Regional Lymph Nodes

The regional lymph nodes are the nodes of the true pelvis, which essentially are the pelvic nodes below the bifurcation of the common iliac arteries. Laterality does not affect the N classification.

## TNM Clinical Classification

*T – Primary Tumour*

The suffix (m) should be added to the appropriate T category to indicate multiple tumours. The suffix (is) may be added to any T to indicate presence of associated carcinoma in situ.

TX      Primary tumour cannot be assessed
T0      No evidence of primary tumour

---

[1] Sobin LH, Wittekind Ch (eds) (1997) TNM classification of malignant tumours, 5th edition. Wiley, New York.

| Ta | Non-invasive papillary carcinoma |
|---|---|
| Tis | Carcinoma in situ: "flat tumour" |
| T1 | Tumour invades subepithelial connective tissue |
| T2 | Tumour invades muscle: |
| T2a | Tumour invades superficial muscle (inner half) |
| T2b | Tumour invades deep muscle (outer half) |
| T3 | Tumour invades perivesical tissue: |
| T3a | microscopically |
| T3b | macroscopically (extravesical mass) |
| T4 | Tumour invades any of the following: prostate, uterus, vagina, pelvic wall, abdominal wall |
| T4a | Tumour invades prostate or uterus or vagina |
| T4b | Tumour invades pelvic wall or abdominal wall |

*N – Regional Lymph Nodes*

| NX | Regional lymph nodes cannot be assessed |
|---|---|
| N0 | No regional lymph node metastasis |
| N1 | Metastasis in a single lymph node 2 cm or less in greatest dimension |
| N2 | Metastasis in a single lymph node more than 2 cm, but not more than 5 cm in greatest dimension, or multiple lymph nodes, none more than 5 cm in greatest dimension |
| N3 | Metastasis in a lymph node more than 5 cm in greatest dimension |

*M – Distant Metastasis*

| MX | Distant metastasis cannot be assessed |
|---|---|
| M0 | No distant metastasis |
| M1 | Distant metastasis |

## pTNM Pathological Classification

The pT, pN and pM categories correspond to the T, N and M categories.

*G – Histopathological Grading*

| | |
|---|---|
| GX | Grade of differentiation cannot be assessed |
| G1 | Well differentiated |
| G2 | Moderately differentiated |
| G3–4 | Poorly differentiated/undifferentiated |

## Stage Grouping

| | | | |
|---|---|---|---|
| Stage 0a | Ta | N0 | M0 |
| Stage 0is | Tis | N0 | M0 |
| Stage I | T1 | N0 | M0 |
| Stage II | T2a | N0 | M0 |
| | T2b | N0 | M0 |
| Stage III | T3a | N0 | M0 |
| | T3b | N0 | M0 |
| | T4a | N0 | M0 |
| Stage IV | T4b | N0 | M0 |
| | Any T | N1, 2, 3 | M0 |
| | Any T | Any N | M1 |

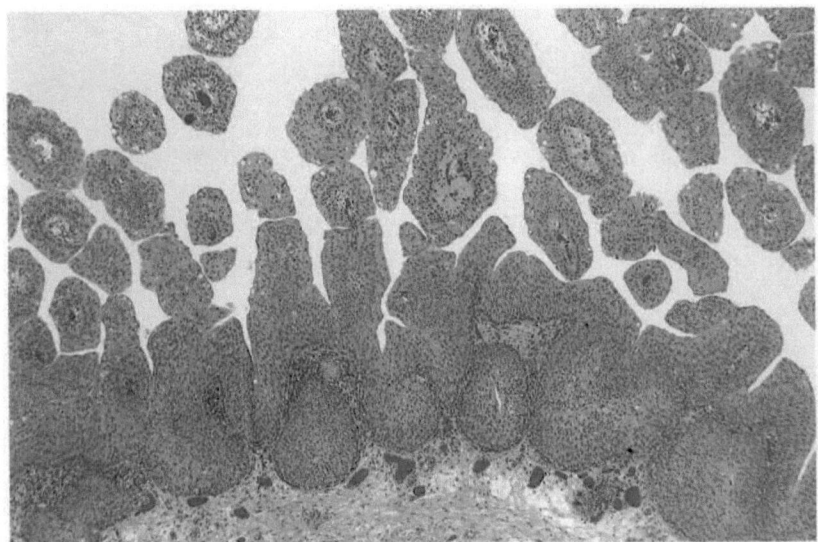

**Fig. 1.** *Urothelial papilloma*

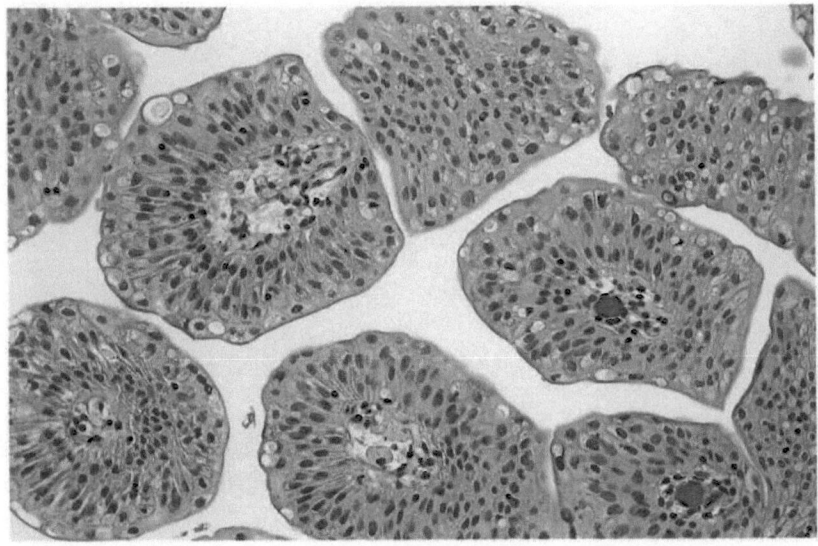

**Fig. 2.** *Urothelial papilloma*

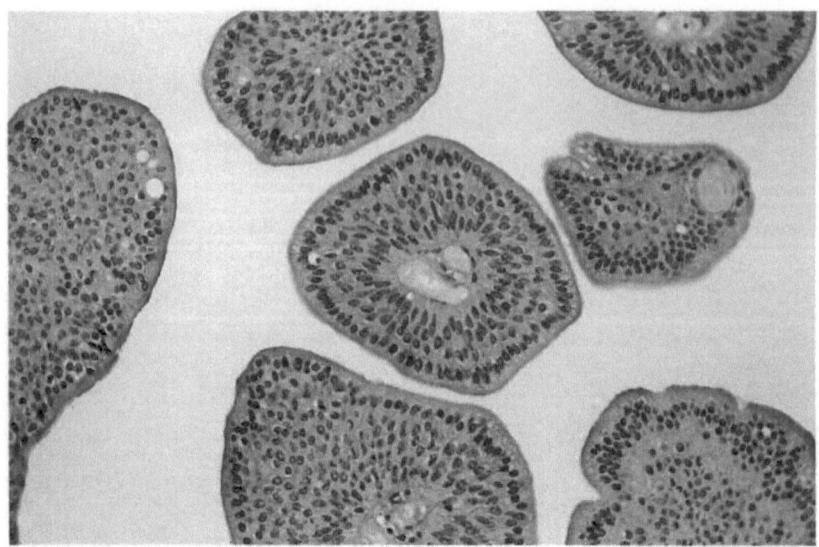

**Fig. 3.** *Urothelial papilloma*

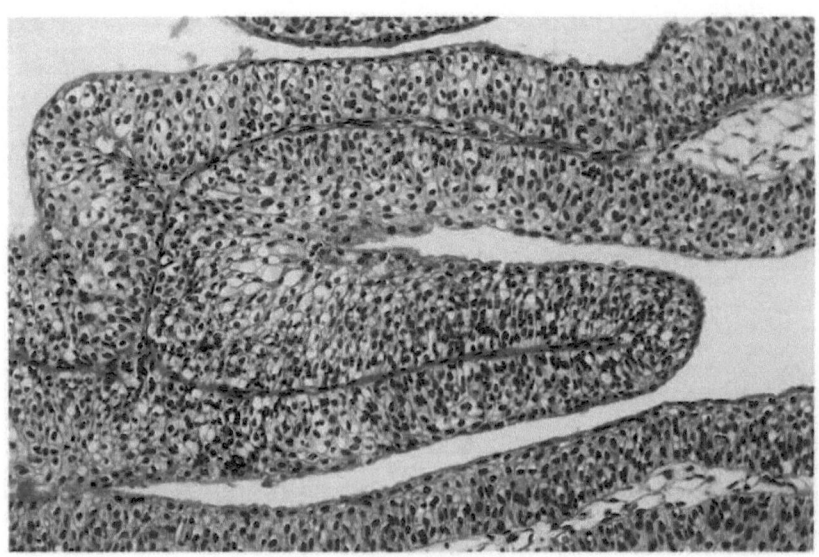

**Fig. 4.** *Urothelial papilloma*

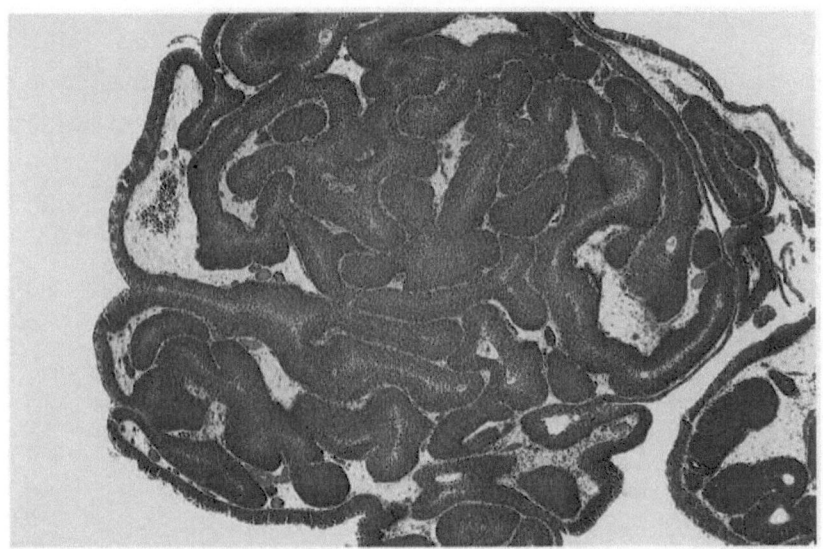

**Fig. 5.** *Urothelial papilloma, inverted type*

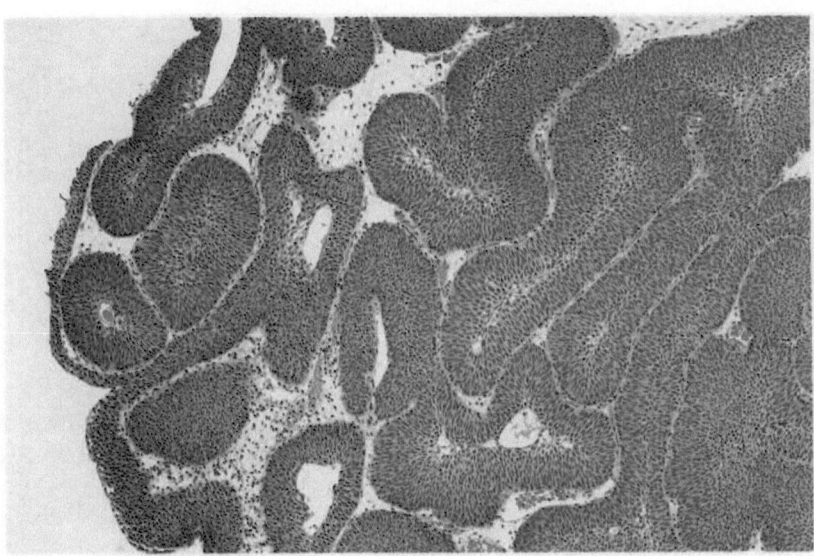

**Fig. 6.** *Urothelial papilloma, inverted type*

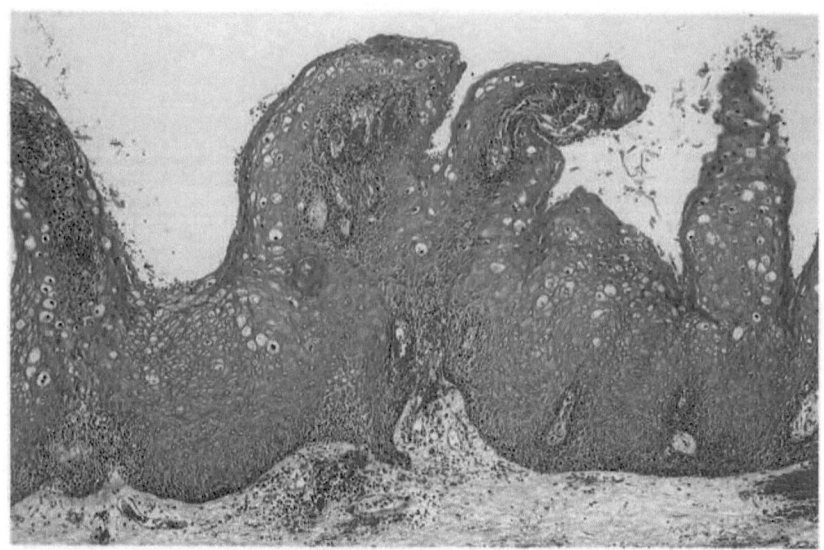

**Fig. 7.** *Squamous cell papilloma (condyloma acuminatum)*

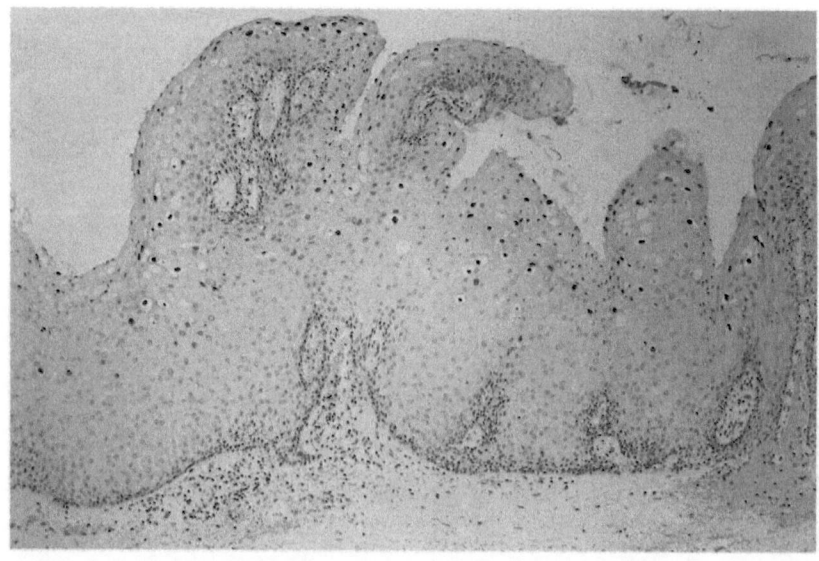

**Fig. 8.** *Squamous cell papilloma.* Human papilloma virus types 6/11, same field as Fig. 7

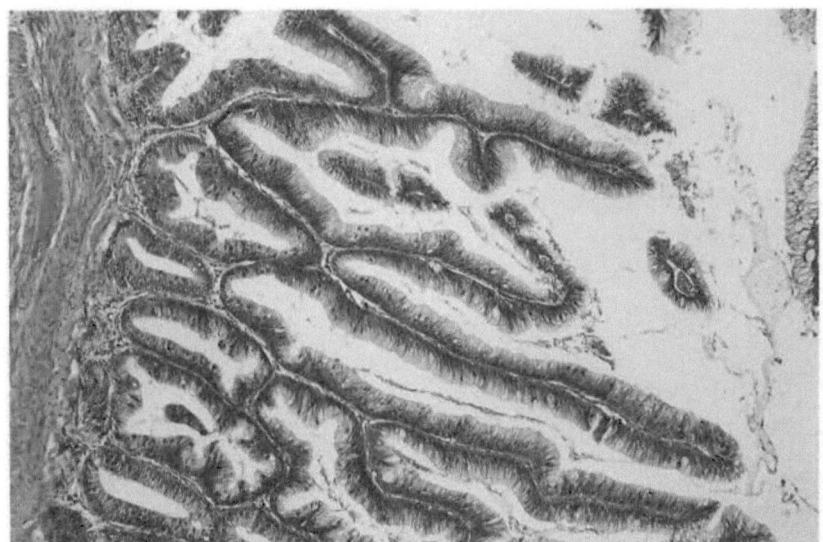

**Fig. 9.** *Villous adenoma*

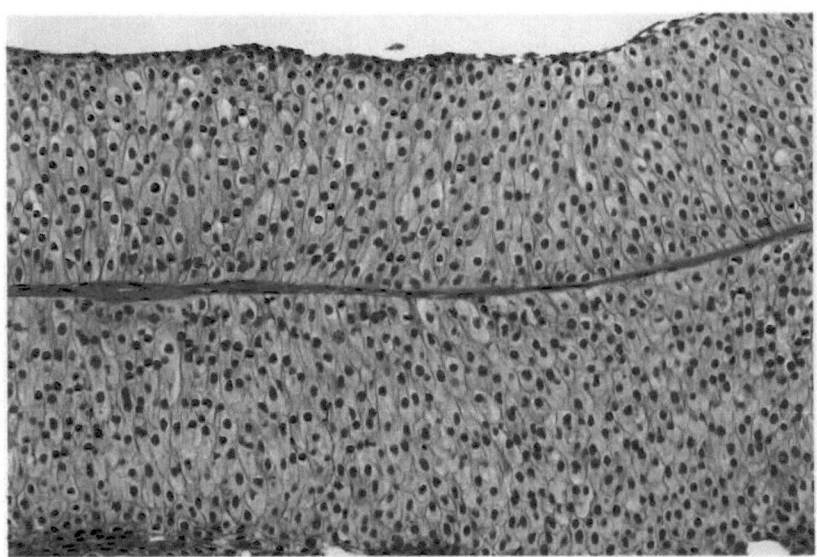

**Fig. 10.** *Papillary urothelial neoplasm of low malignant potential.* The epithelium is thicker than that of the papilloma, but the cells are normal

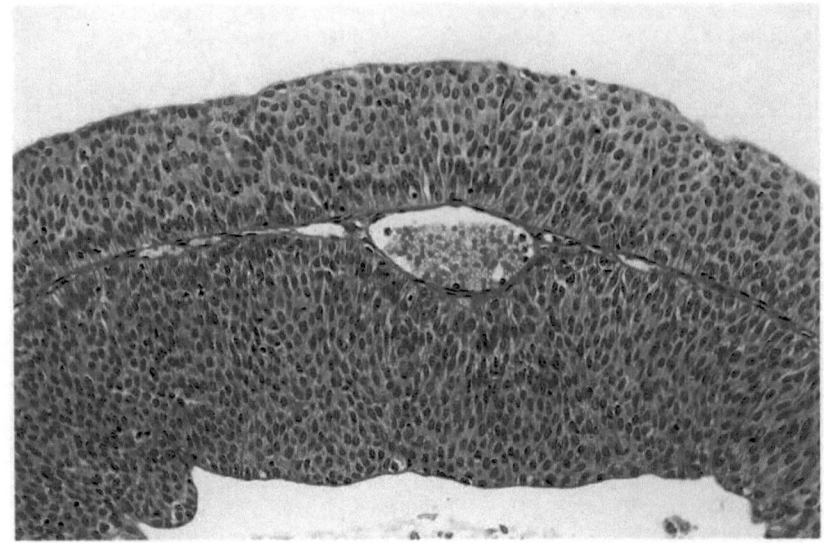

**Fig. 11.** *Papillary urothelial neoplasm of low malignant potential.* There is minimal variation of architectural and nuclear features

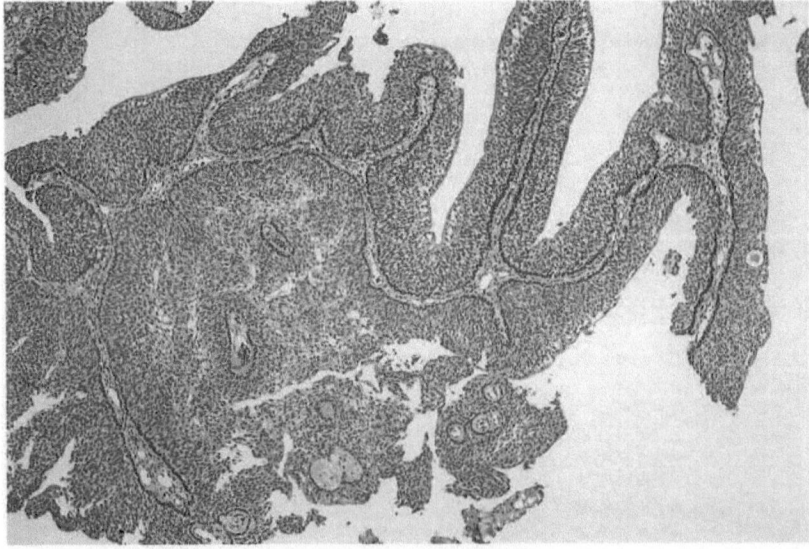

**Fig. 12.** *Papillary urothelial neoplasm of low malignant potential.* There is a prominent inverted growth pattern

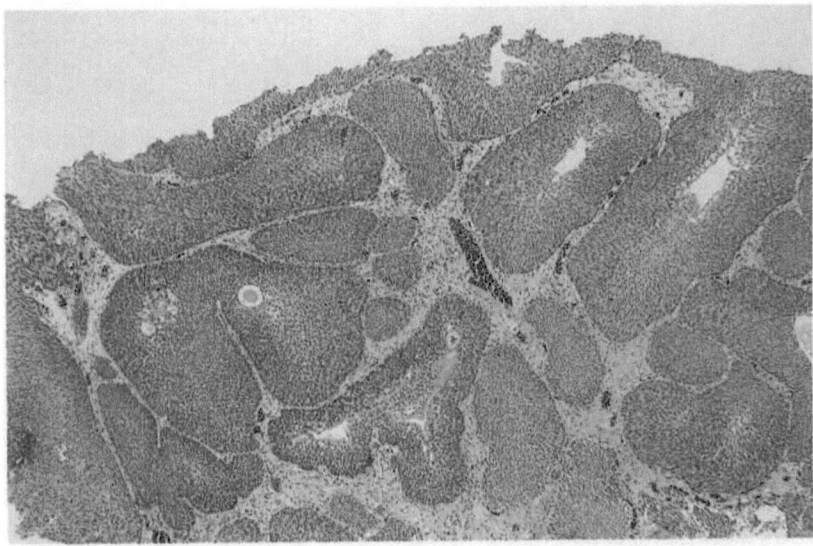

**Fig. 13.** *Papillary urothelial carcinoma, inverted pattern grade I.* Same patient as in Fig. 12, 3 years later. Focal mild anaplasia (*bottom centre*) establishes diagnosis of grade I carcinoma

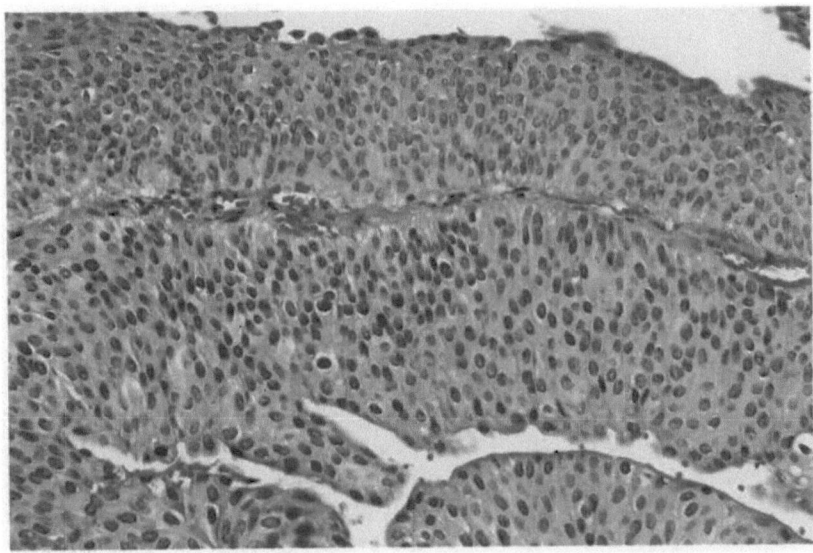

**Fig. 14.** *Papillary urothelial carcinoma, grade I.* The upper side of this frond resembles the neoplasm of low malignant potential. The lower side shows variations of nuclear size, staining and crowding

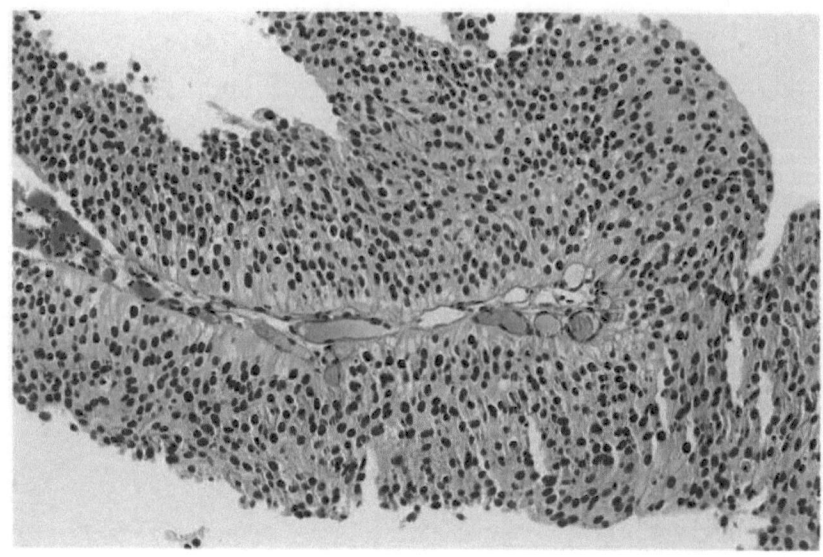

**Fig. 15.** *Papillary urothelial carcinoma, grade I*

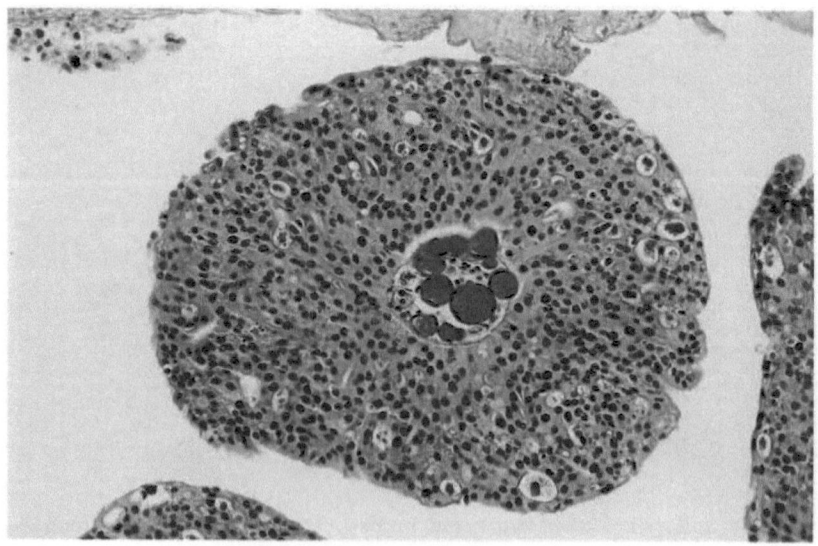

**Fig. 16.** *Papillary urothelial carcinoma, grade I*

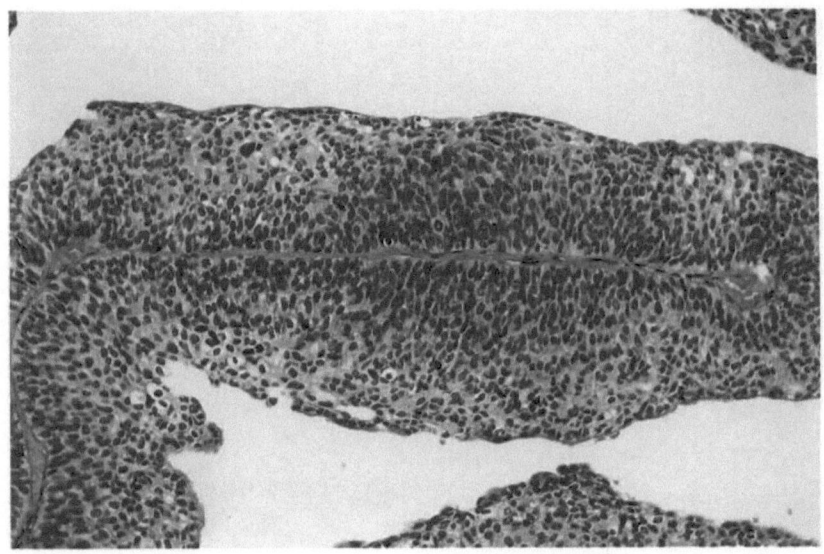

**Fig. 17.** *Papillary urothelial carcinoma, grade II.* Nuclear variation is greater than in grade I tumours, but some polarity is retained

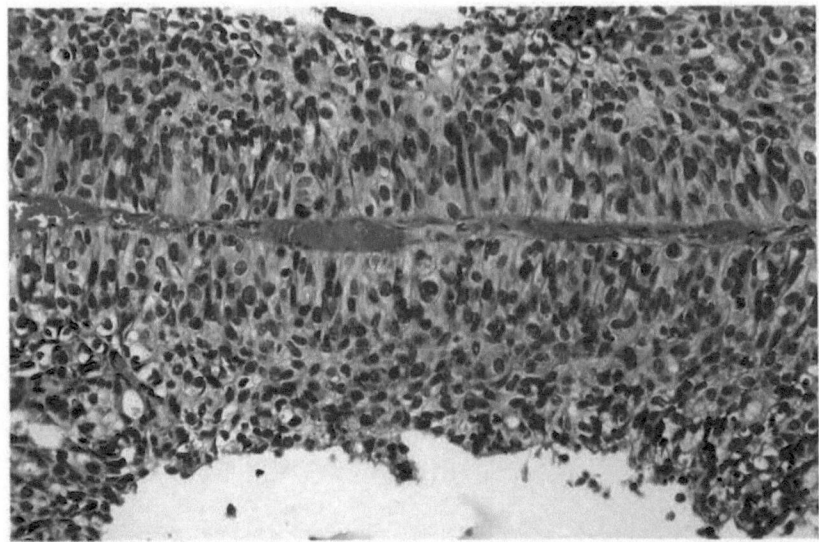

**Fig. 18.** *Papillary urothelial carcinoma, grade II*

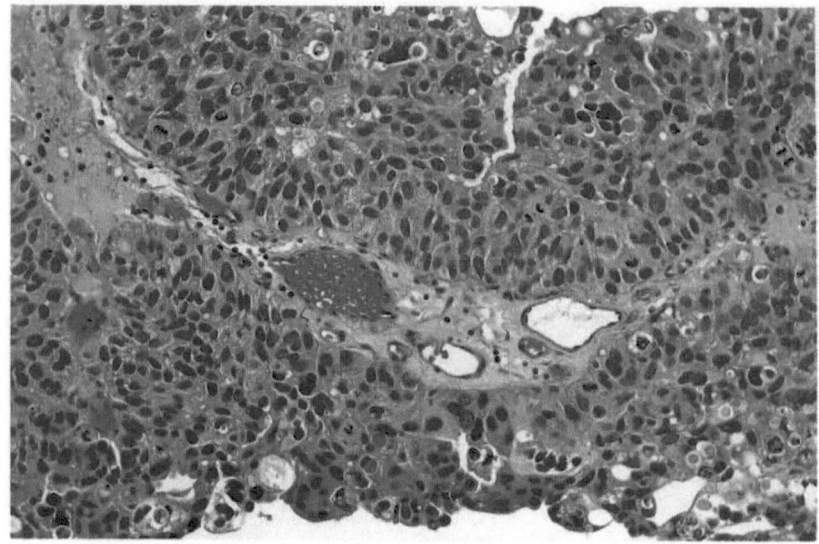

**Fig. 19.** *Papillary urothelial carcinoma, grade III.* There is marked variation of all nuclear parameters and an absence of polarity

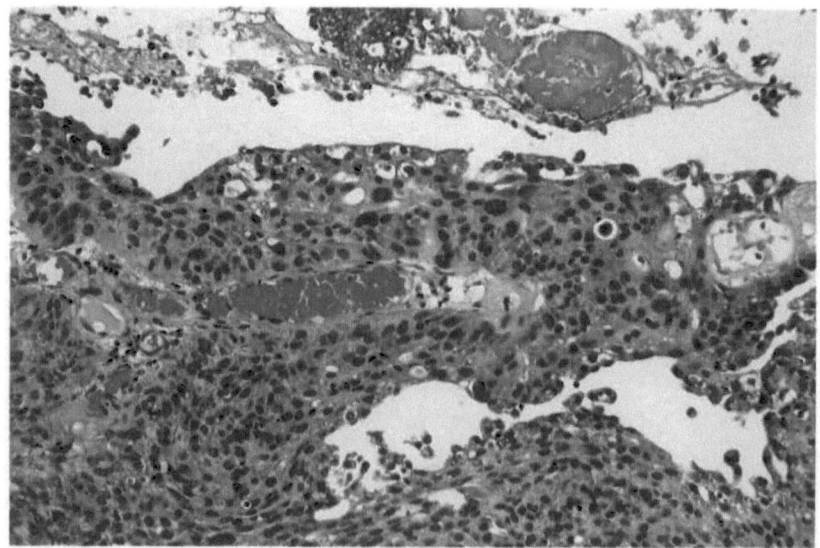

**Fig. 20.** *Papillary urothelial carcinoma, grade III*

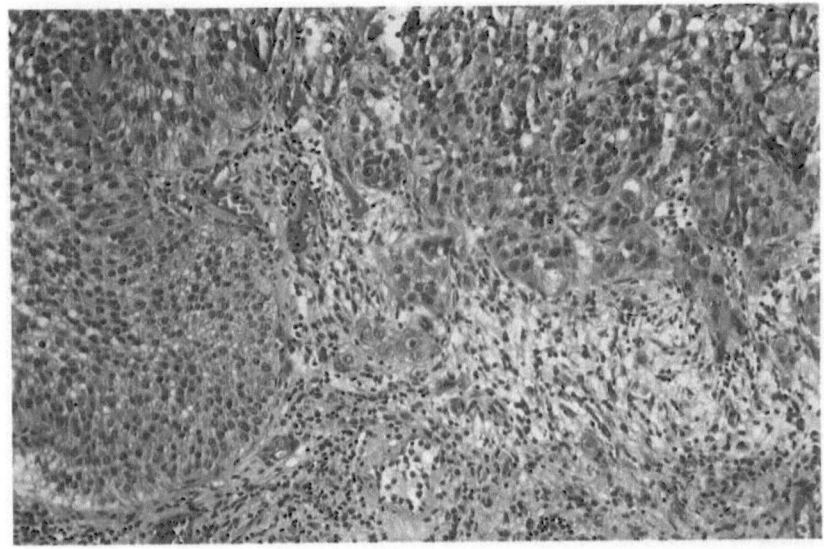

**Fig. 21.** *Urothelial carcinoma* infiltrating lamina propria. Note altered character of stroma adjacent to invasive lesion (*right*) compared to non-invasive area (*left*)

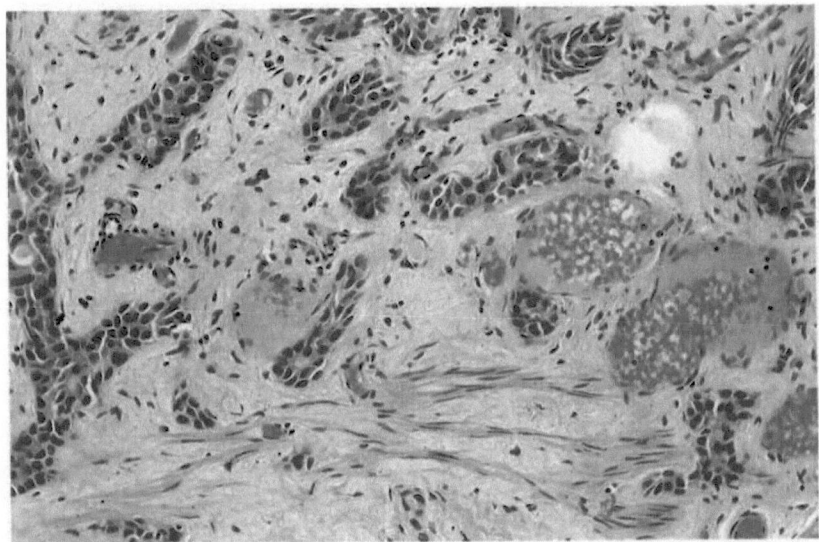

**Fig. 22.** *Urothelial carcinoma* invading muscularis mucosae

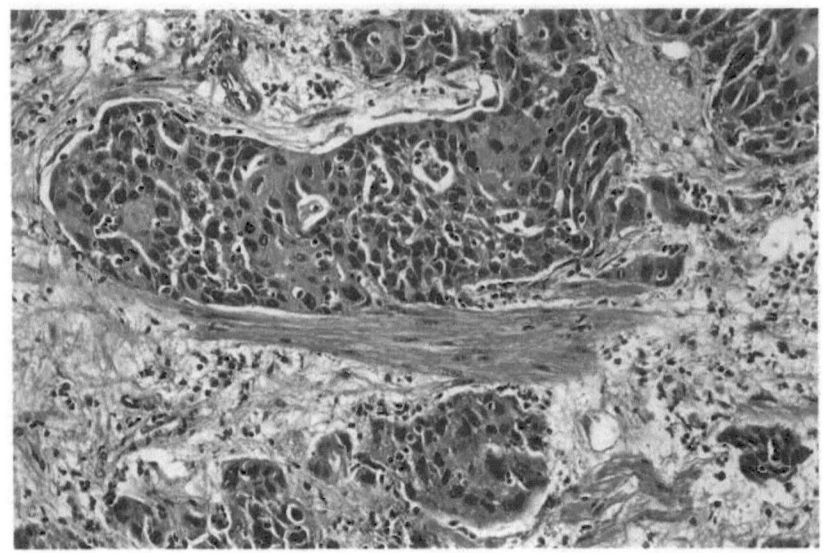

**Fig. 23.** *Urothelial carcinoma* invading muscularis mucosae

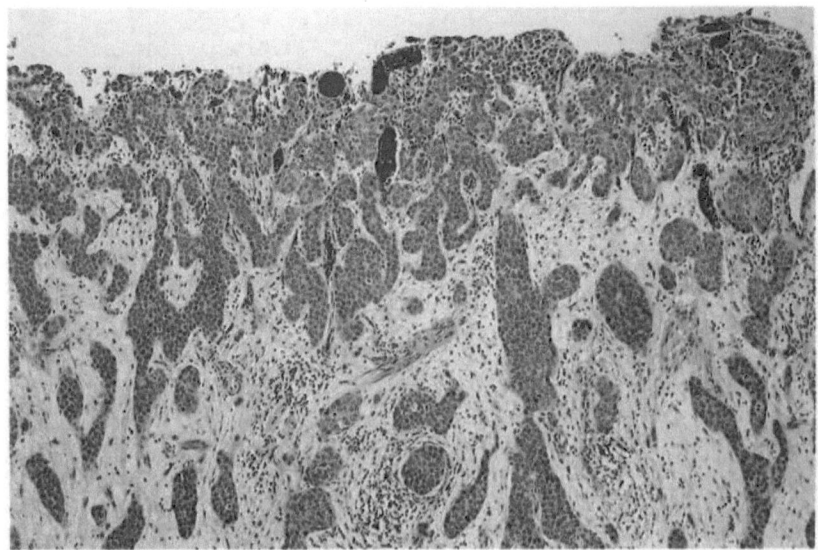

**Fig. 24.** *Urothelial carcinoma.* Tentacular growth pattern

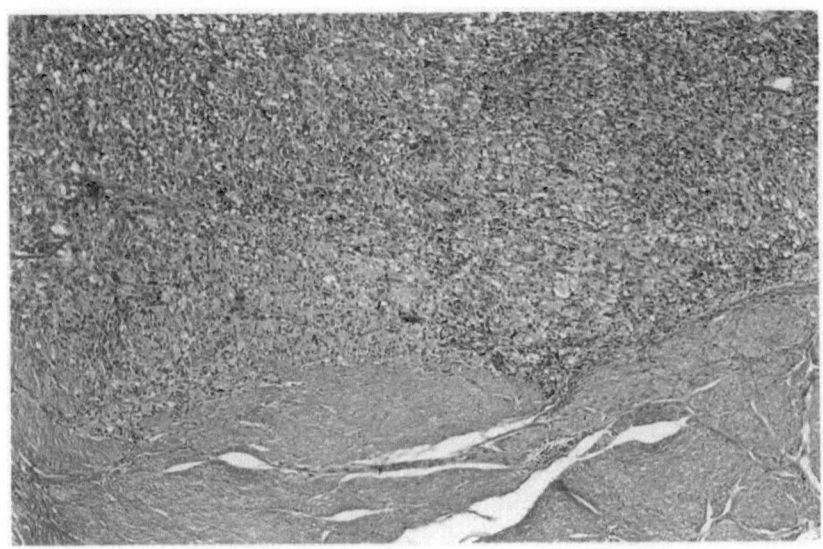

**Fig. 25.** *Urothelial carcinoma.* Broad-front, pushing margins

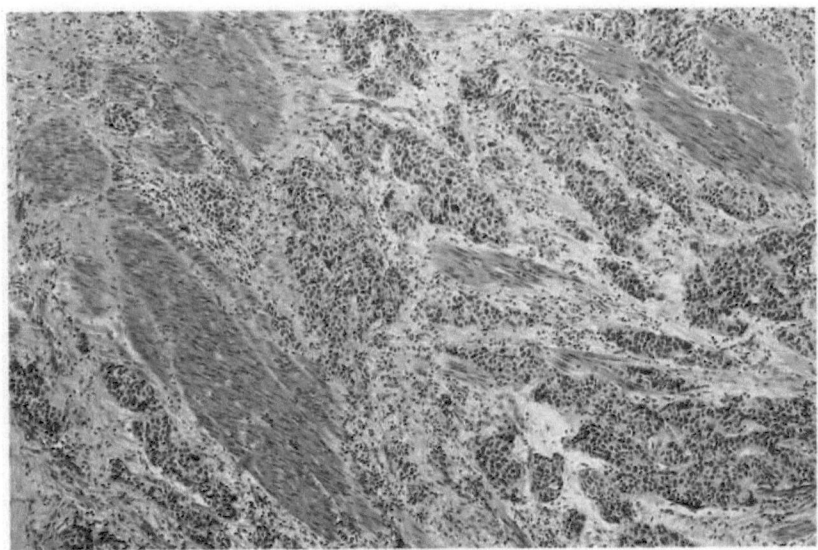

**Fig. 26.** *Urothelial carcinoma* invading muscularis propria

46

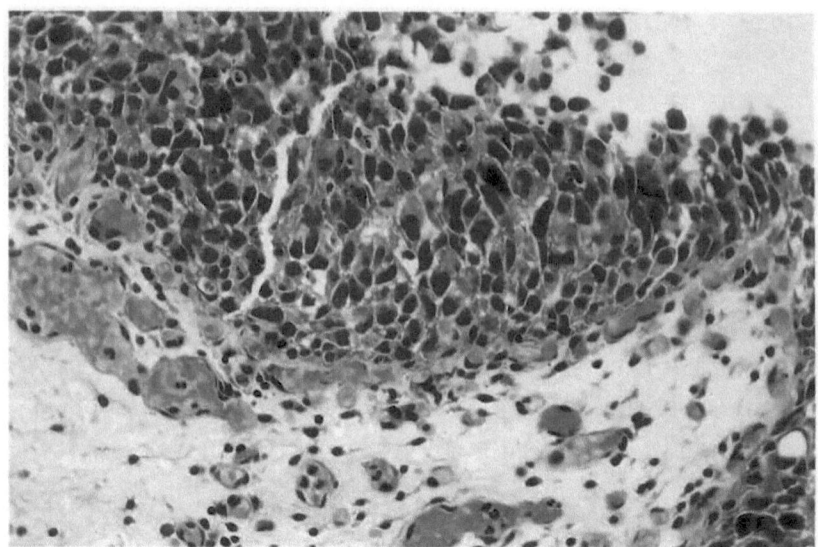

**Fig. 27.** *Carcinoma in situ*

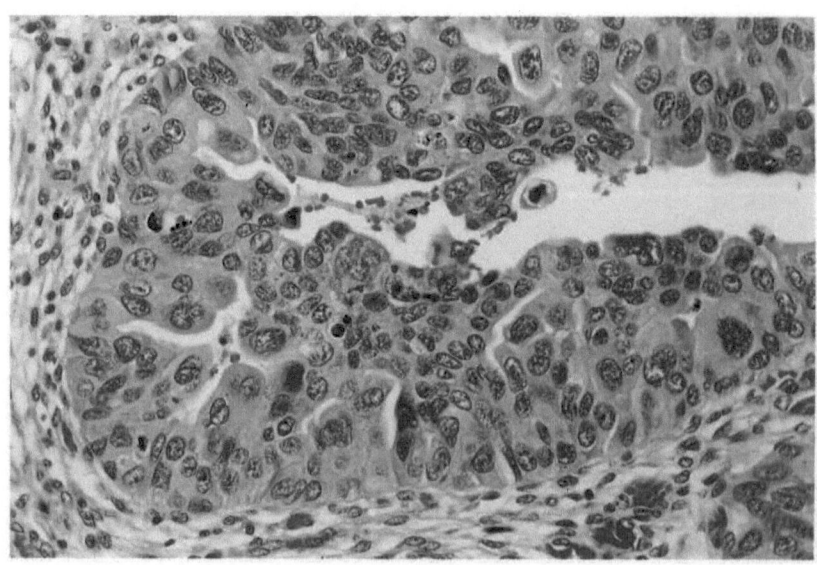

**Fig. 28.** *Carcinoma in situ*

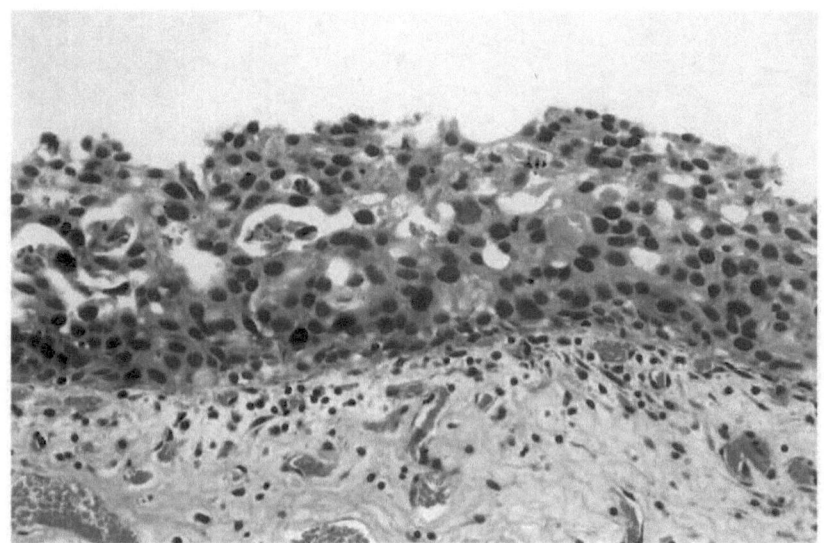

**Fig. 29.** *Carcinoma in situ*

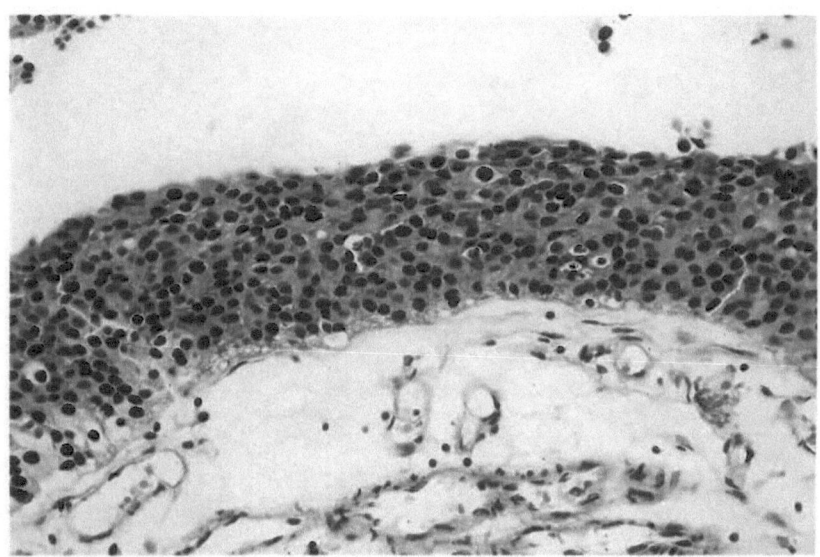

**Fig. 30.** *Carcinoma in situ*

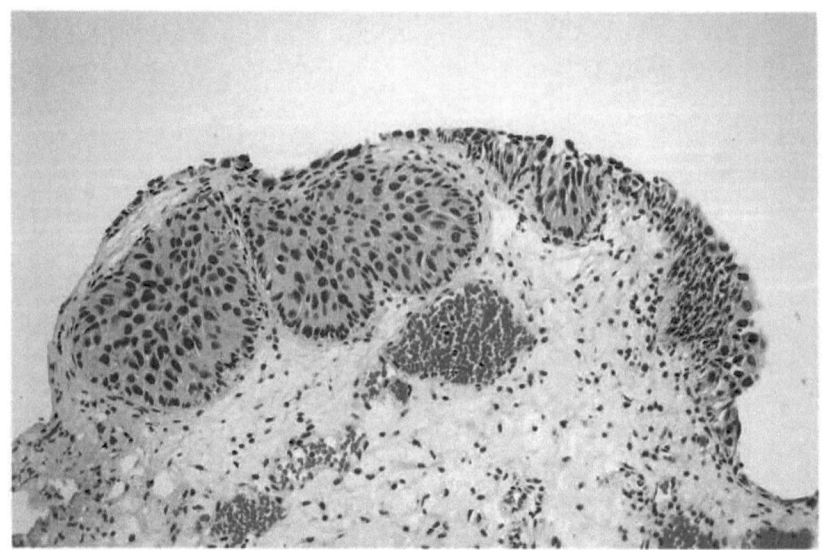

**Fig. 31.** *Carcinoma in situ* involving von Brunn nests

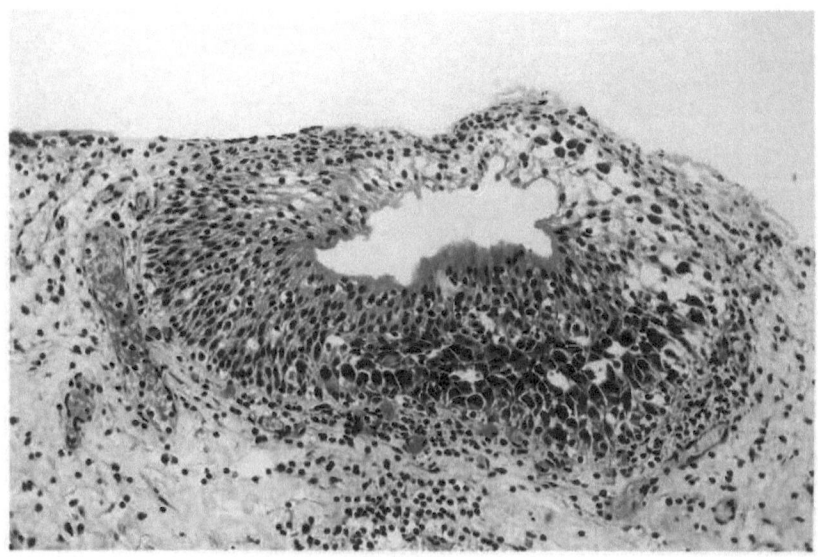

**Fig. 32.** *Carcinoma in situ* involving cystitis cystica

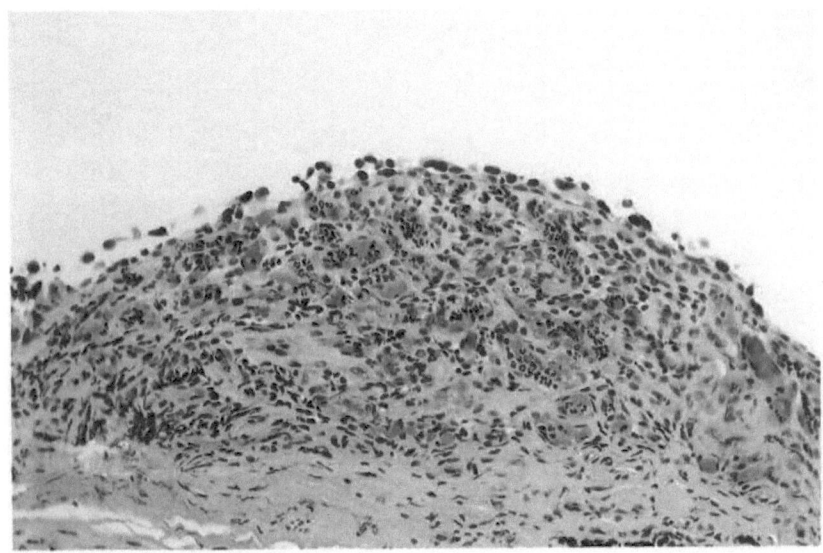

**Fig. 33.** *Carcinoma in situ*

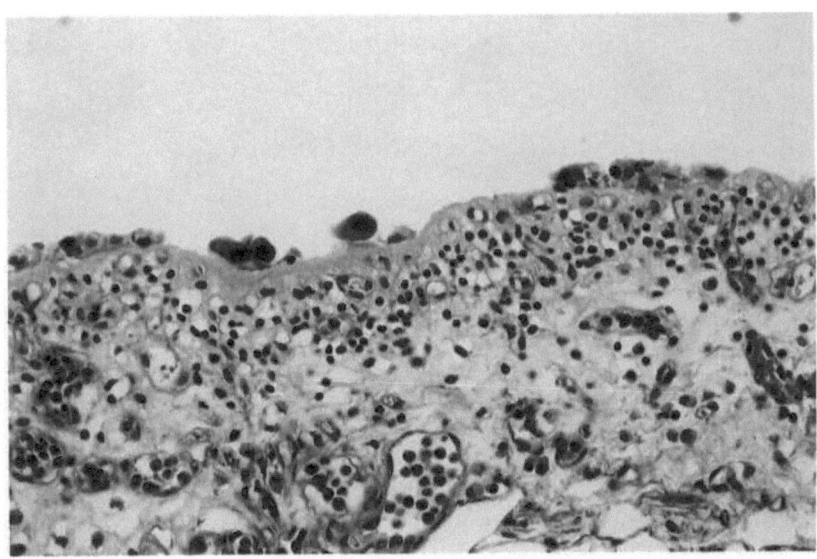

**Fig. 34.** *Carcinoma in situ*

50

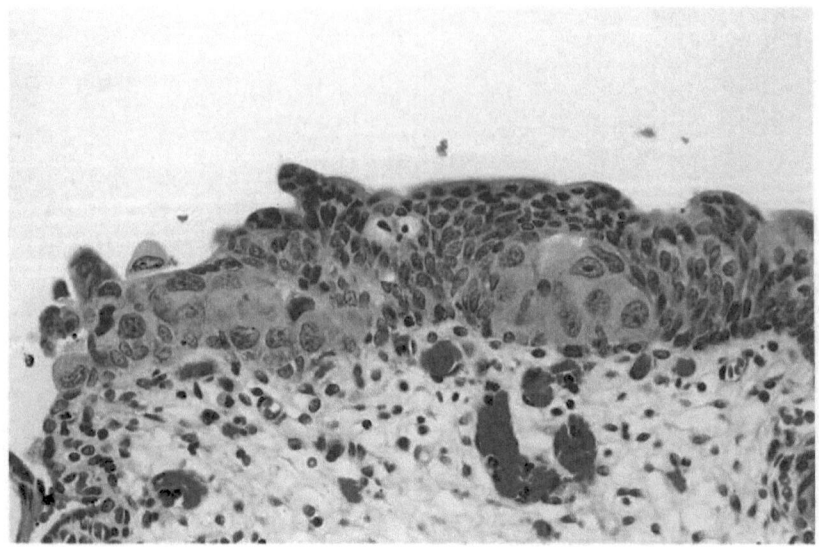

**Fig. 35.** *Carcinoma in situ, pagetoid*

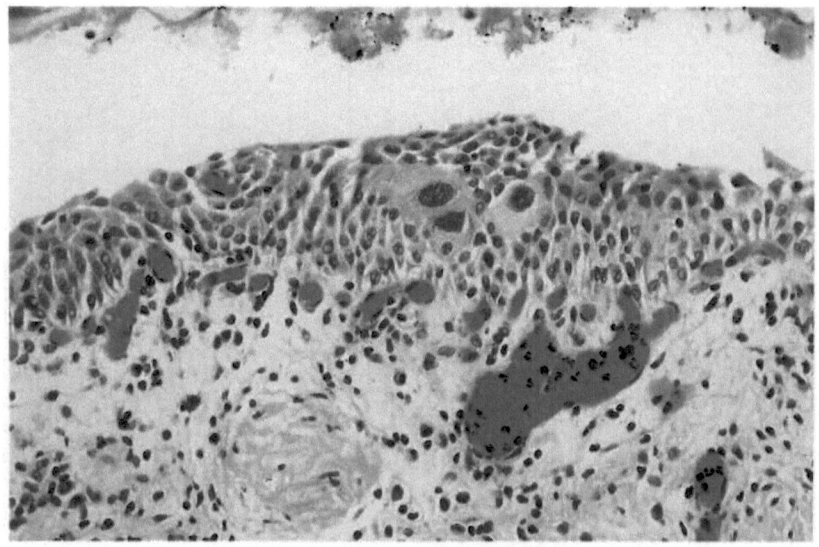

**Fig. 36.** *Carcinoma in situ, pagetoid*

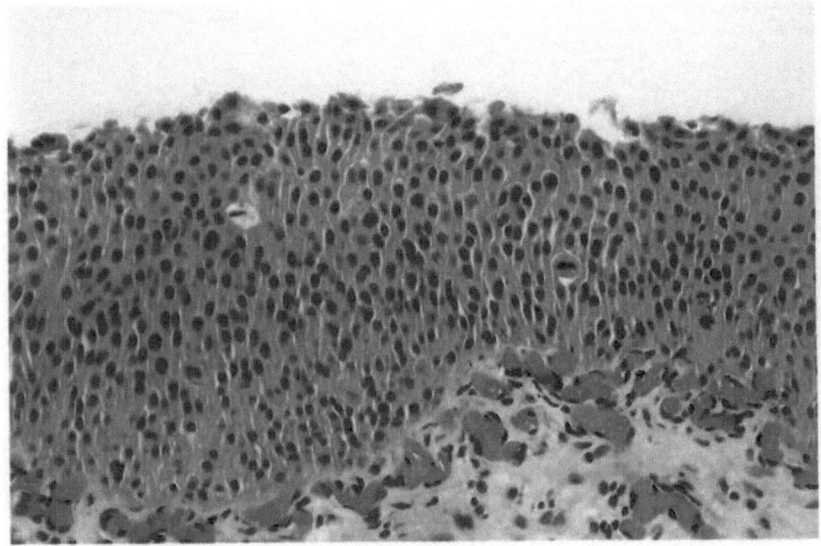

**Fig. 37.** *Atypia (or dysplasia).* Neoplastic epithelium with changes insufficient for a diagnosis of carcinoma in situ

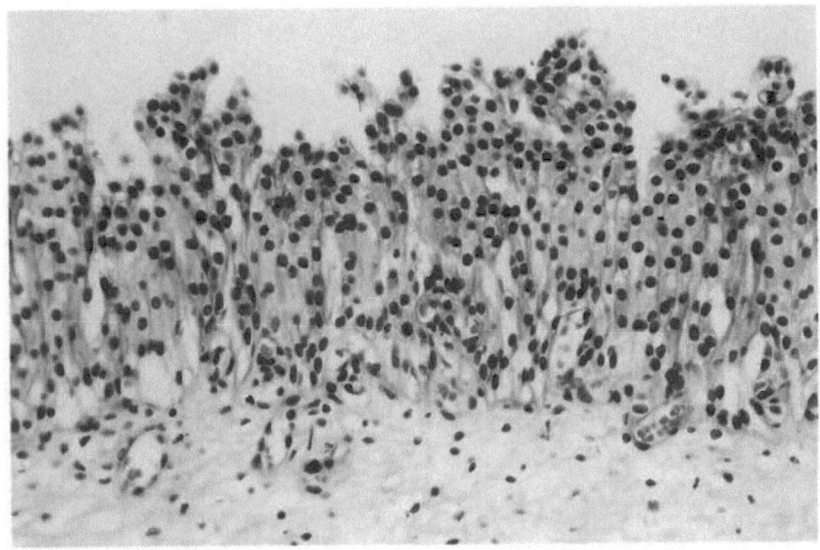

**Fig. 38.** *Atypia (or dysplasia)*

52

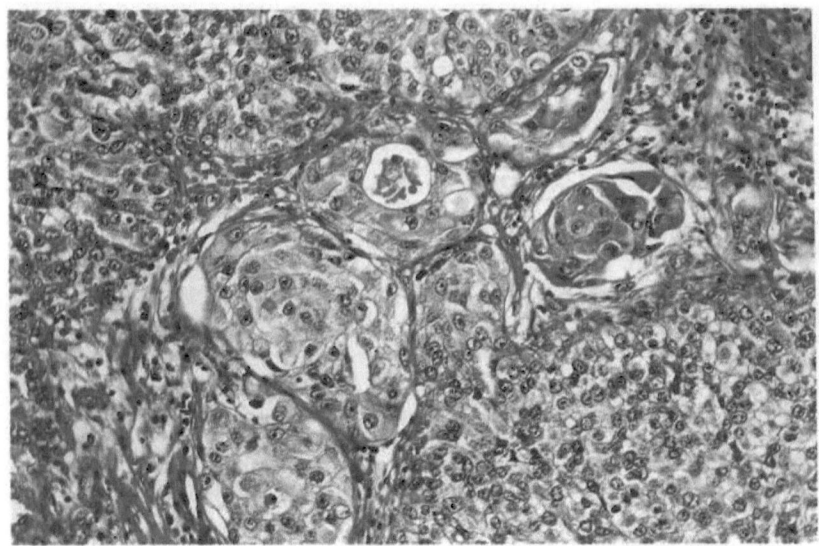

**Fig. 39.** *Urothelial carcinoma with squamous metaplasia*

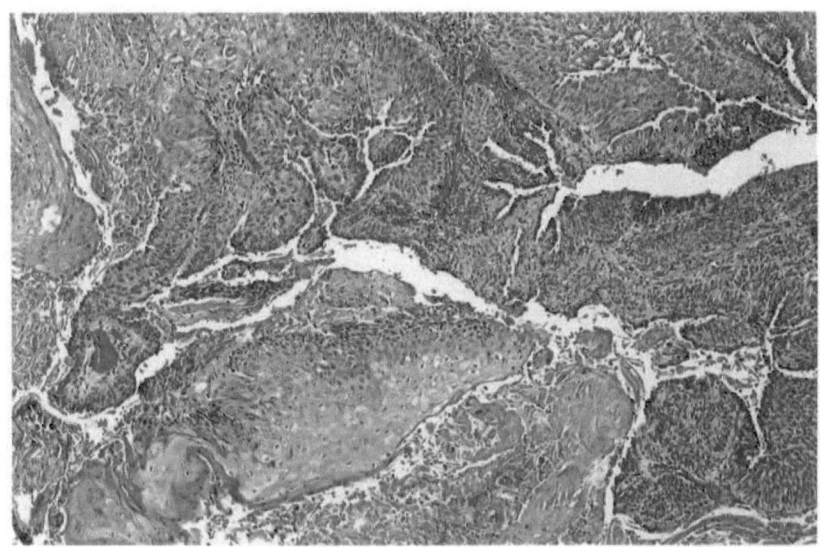

**Fig. 40.** *Urothelial carcinoma with squamous metaplasia*

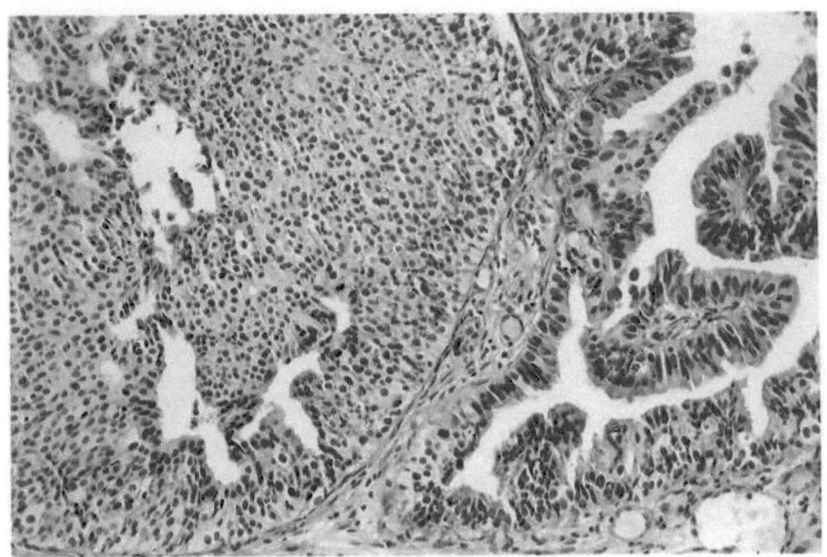

**Fig. 41.** *Urothelial carcinoma with glandular metaplasia*

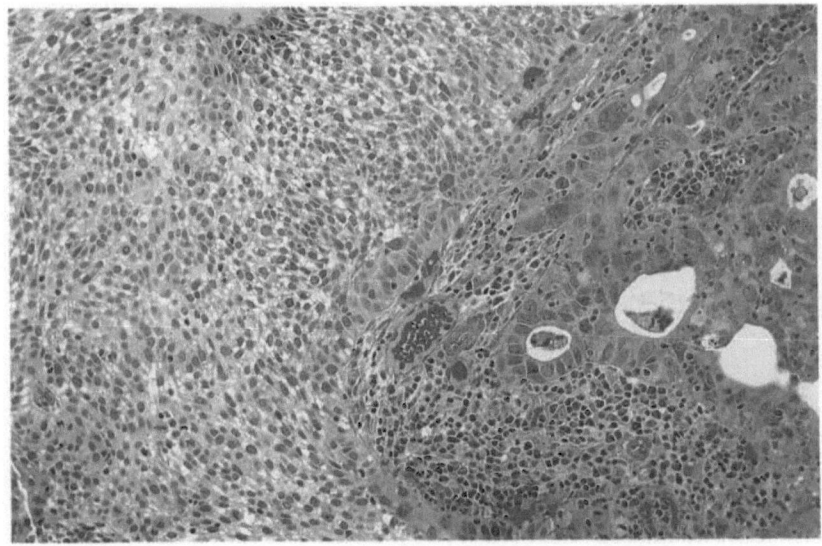

**Fig. 42.** *Urothelial carcinoma with glandular metaplasia*

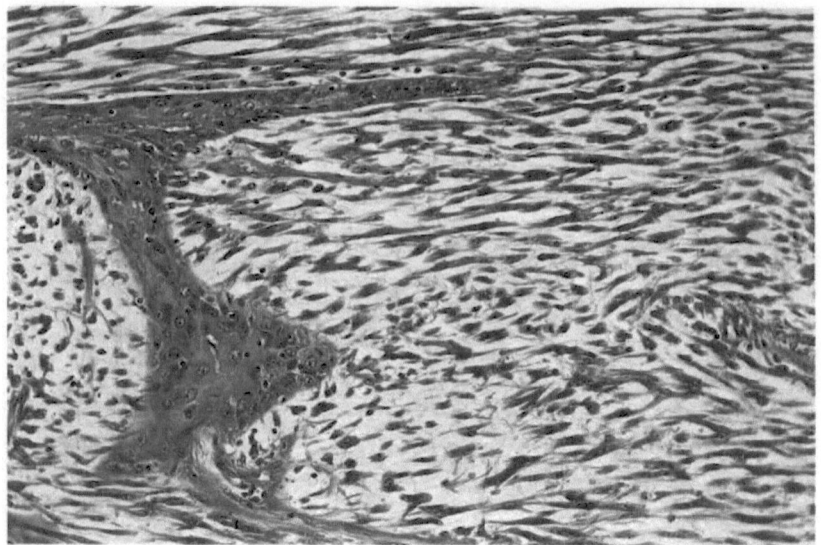

**Fig. 43.** *Spindle cell carcinoma*

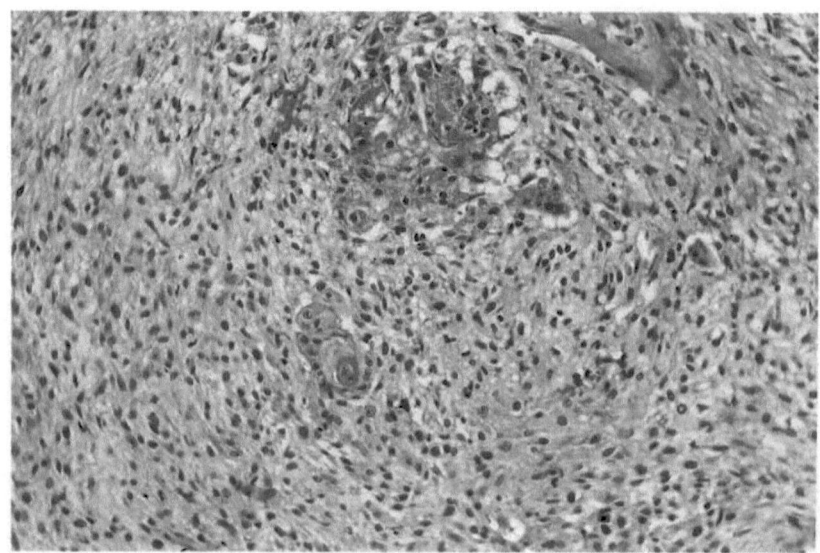

**Fig. 44.** *Spindle cell carcinoma.* Differentiated areas of squamous cell carcinoma

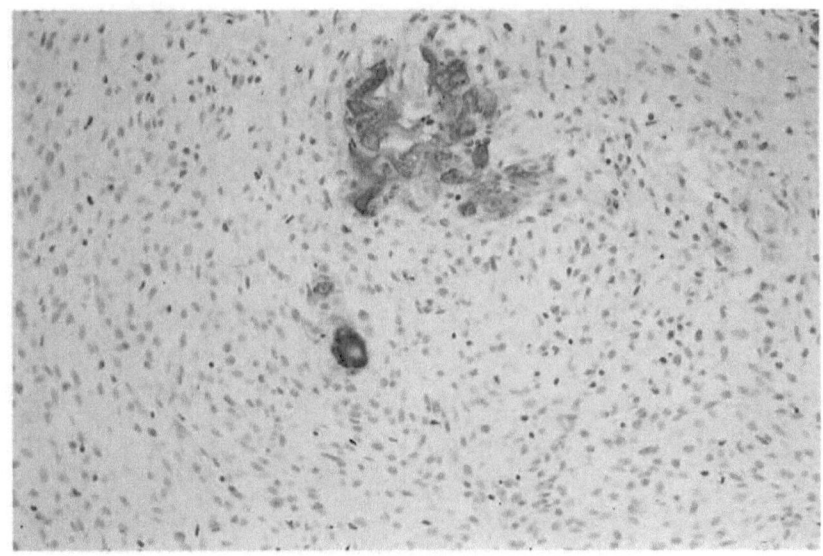

**Fig. 45.** *Spindle cell carcinoma.* Cytokeratin, same field as Fig. 44

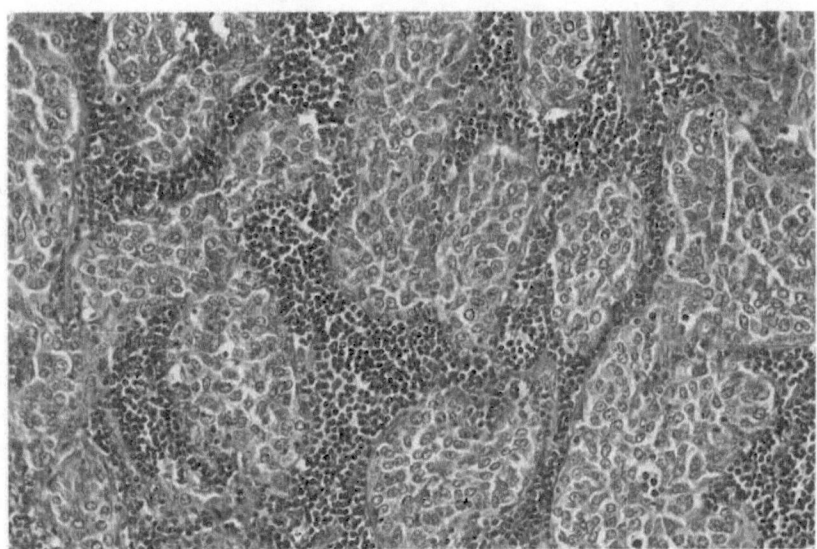

**Fig. 46.** *Urothelial carcinoma with lymphocytic infiltrate*

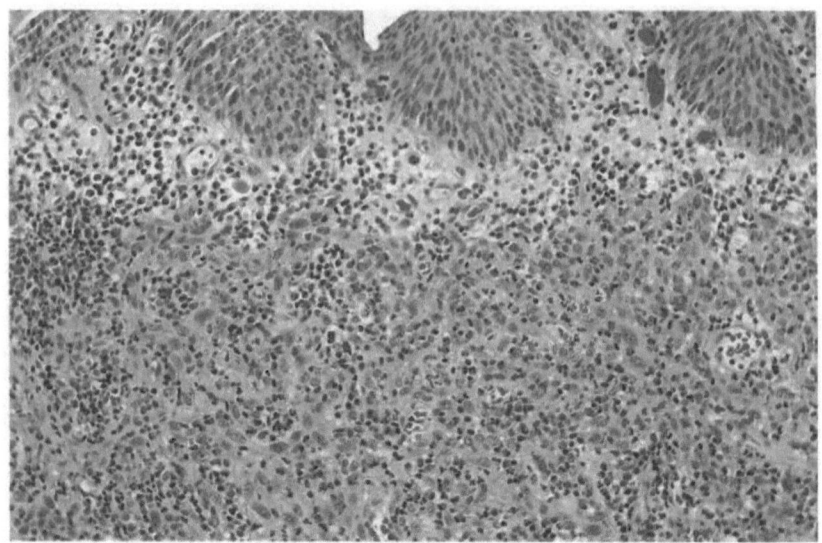

**Fig. 47.** *Urothelial carcinoma with lymphocytic infiltrate, lymphoepithelioma-like variant*

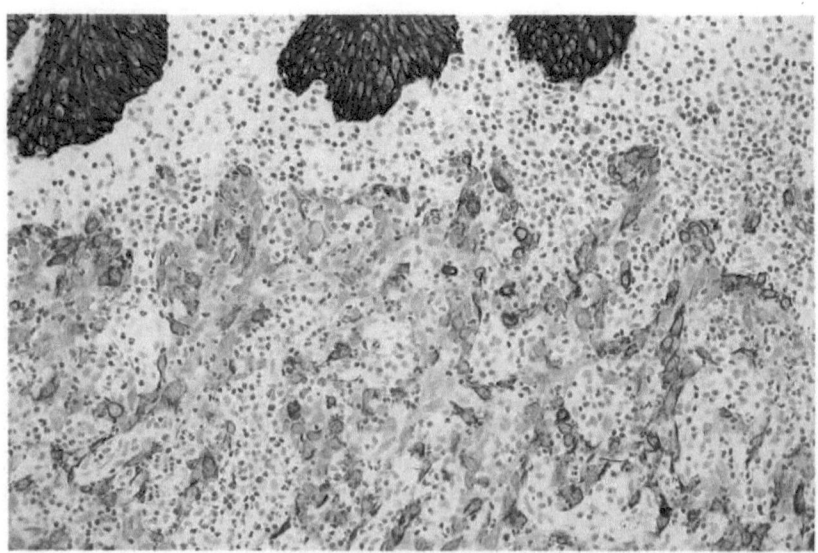

**Fig. 48.** *Urothelial carcinoma with lymphocytic infiltrate, lymphoepithelioma-like variant.* Cytokeratin, same field as Fig. 47

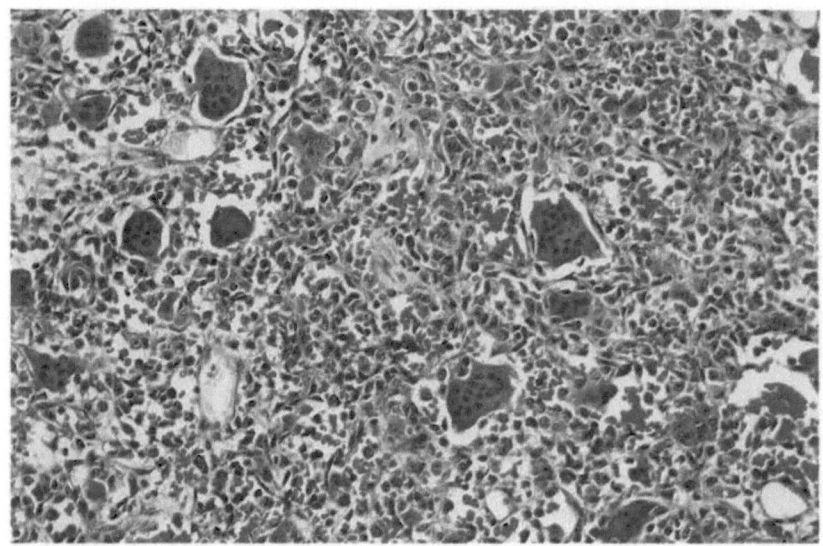

**Fig. 49.** *Urothelial carcinoma, osteoclastic variant.* Urothelial carcinoma was present in other areas of the tumour

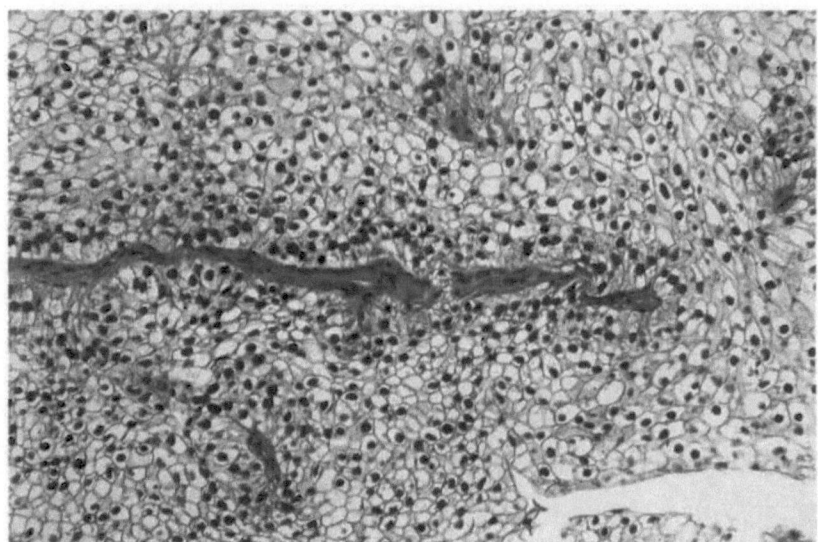

**Fig. 50.** *Urothelial carcinoma, clear cell variant*

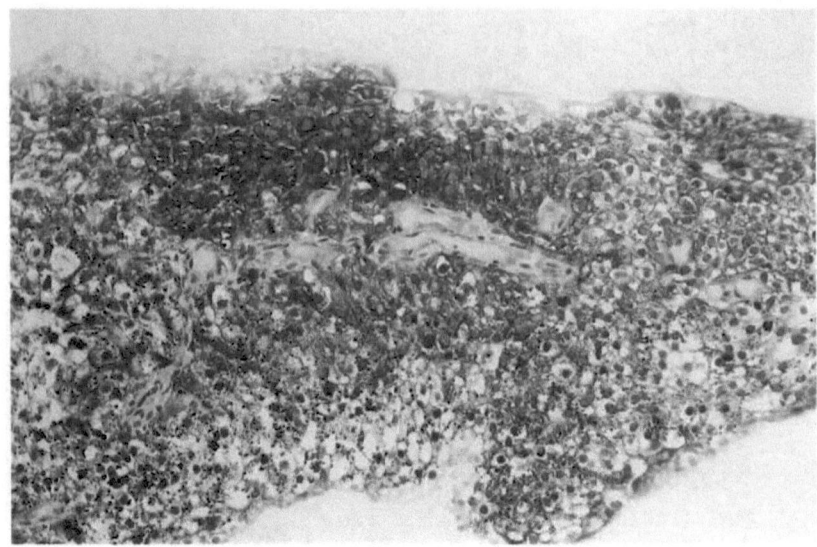

**Fig. 51.** *Urothelial carcinoma, clear cell variant.* Abundant glycogen with the periodic acid–Schiff reaction, same tumour as Fig. 50

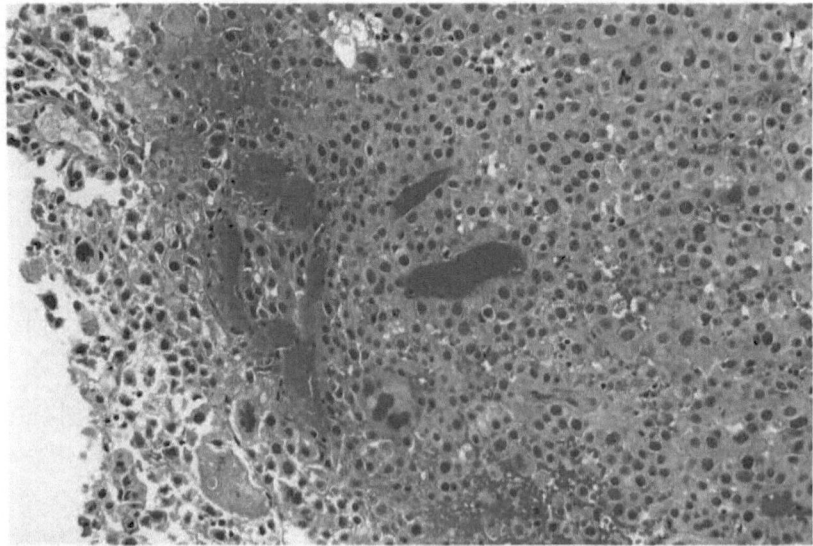

**Fig. 52.** *Urothelial carcinoma with ectopic placental glycoprotein production*

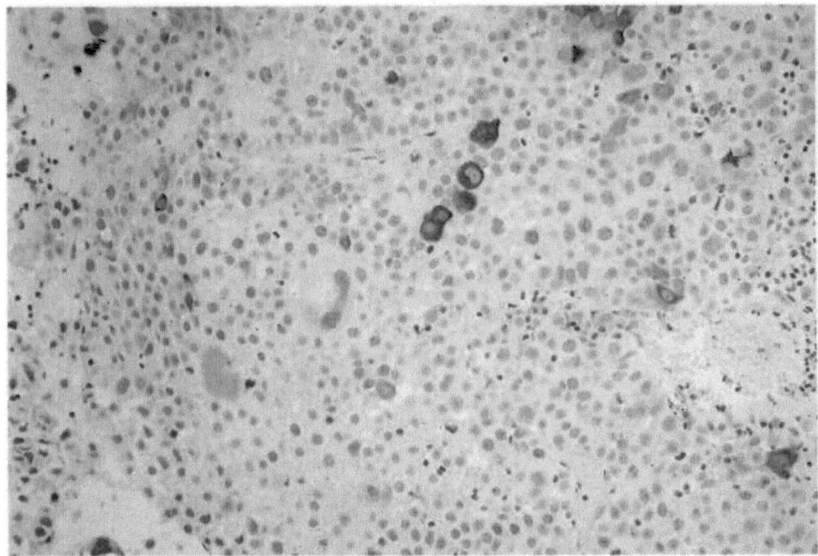

**Fig. 53.** *Urothelial carcinoma with ectopic placental glycoprotein production.* Human chorionic gonadotropin immunostain, same field as Fig. 52. Note that small cells are reactive and large cell is not

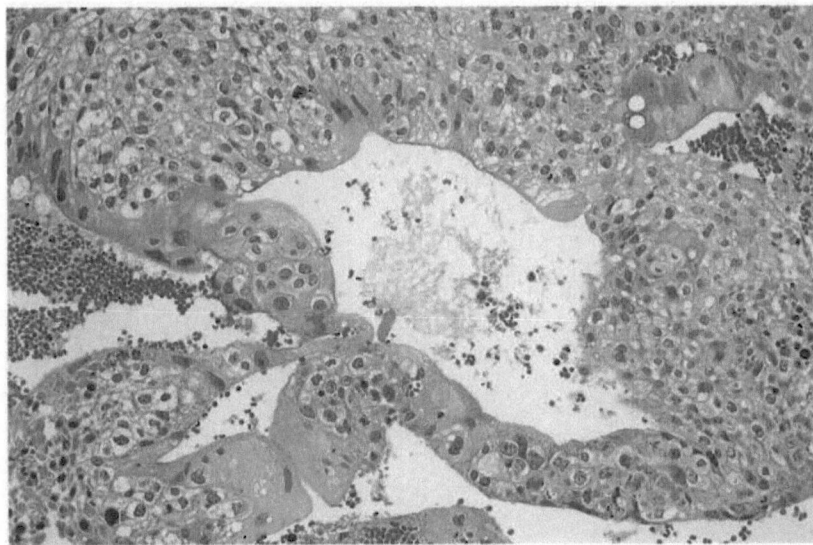

**Fig. 54.** *Urothelial carcinoma with ectopic placental glycoprotein production*

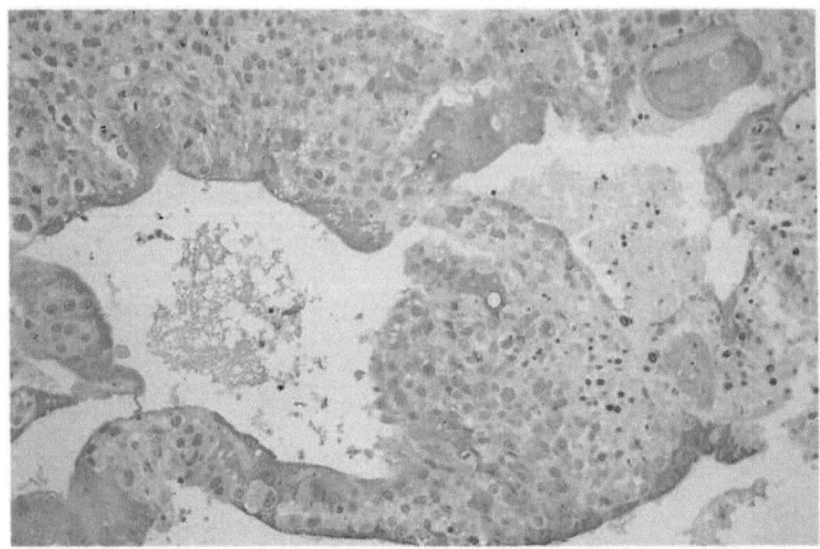

**Fig. 55.** *Urothelial carcinoma with ectopic placental glycoprotein production.* The syncytiotrophoblast-like cells are positive for human chorionic gonadotropin, but, unlike choriocarcinoma, the small cells are also positive. Same field as Fig. 54

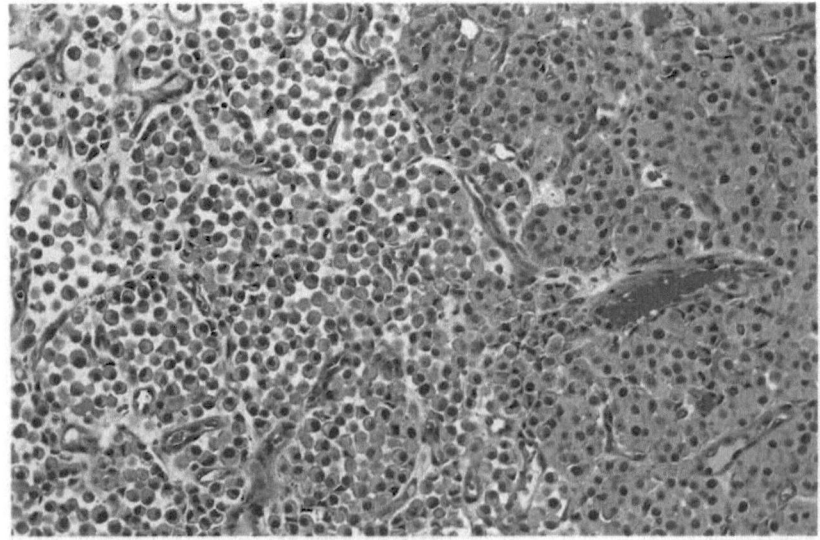

**Fig. 56.** *Urothelial carcinoma, plasmacytoid variant*

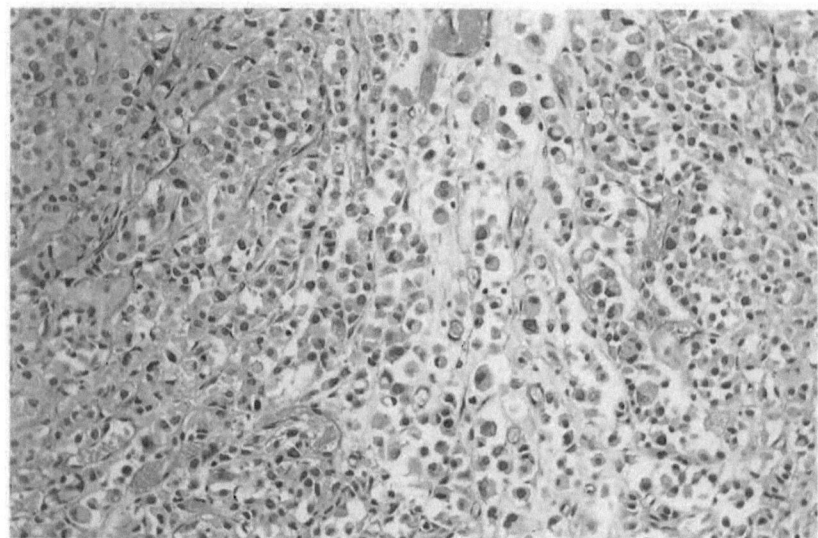

**Fig. 57.** *Urothelial carcinoma, plasmacytoid variant.* Same case as Fig. 56. Note that some cells are mucin-positive with periodic acid–Schiff stain

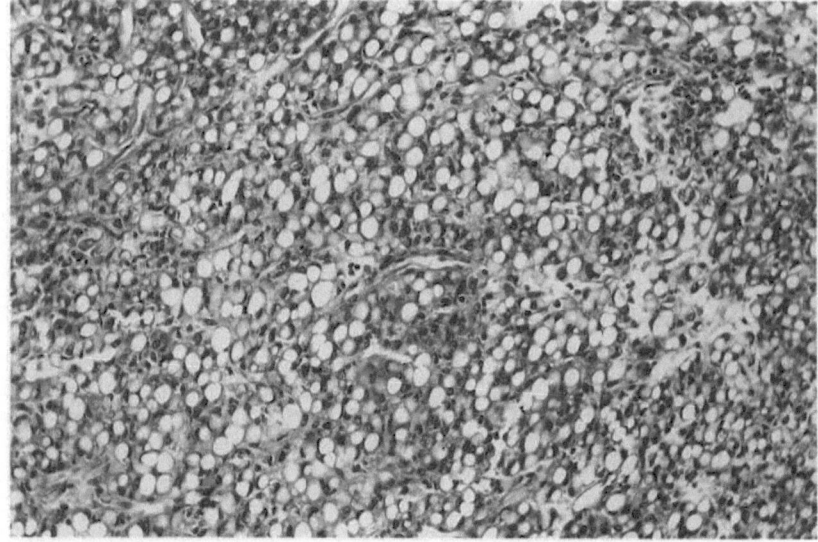

**Fig. 58.** *Urothelial carcinoma, lipid cell variant.* The cells resemble signet-ring li-poblasts

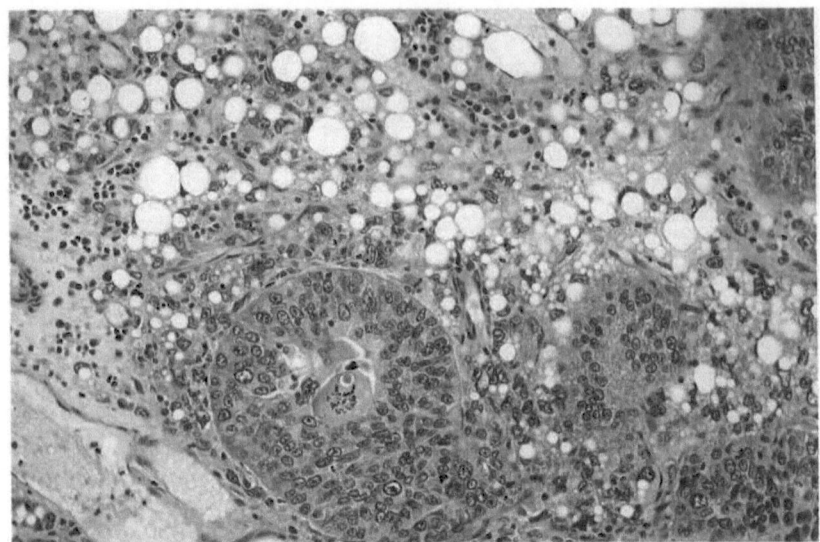

**Fig. 59.** *Urothelial carcinoma, lipid cell variant.* Typical urothelial carcinoma is also present

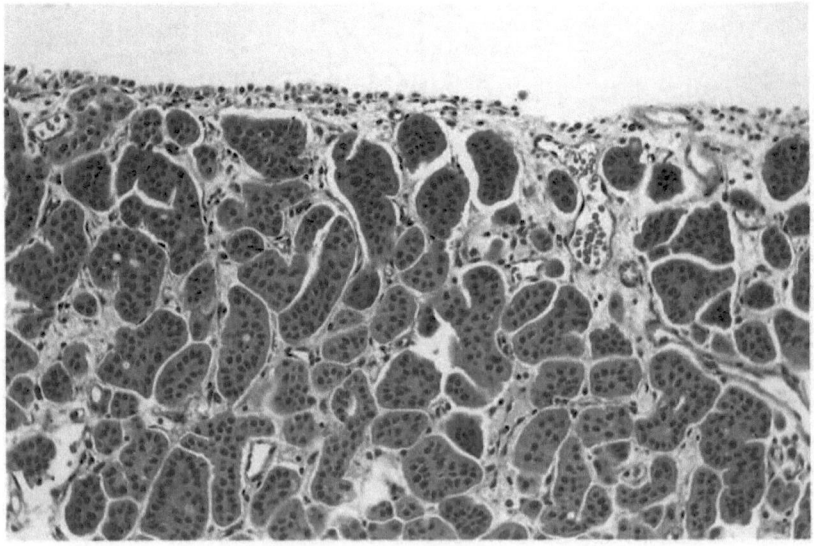

**Fig. 60.** *Urothelial carcinoma, micropapillary variant*

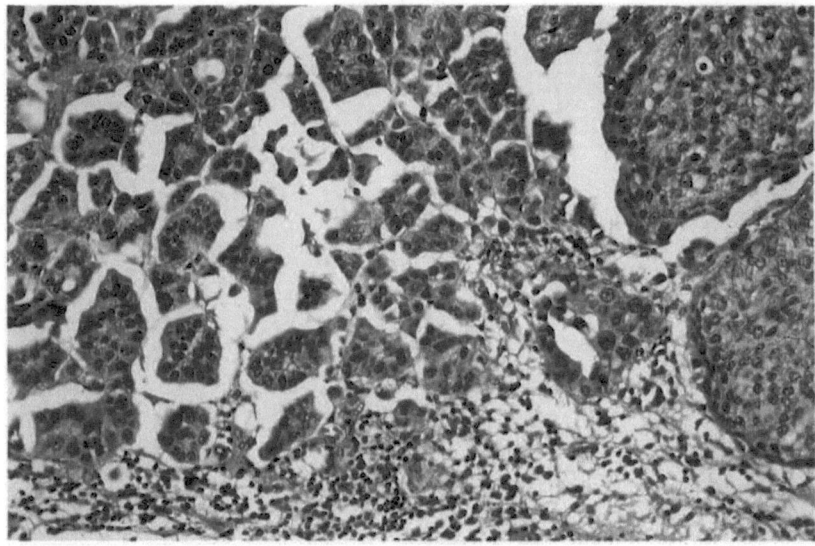

**Fig. 61.** *Urothelial carcinoma, micropapillary variant.* Typical urothelial carcinoma is also present

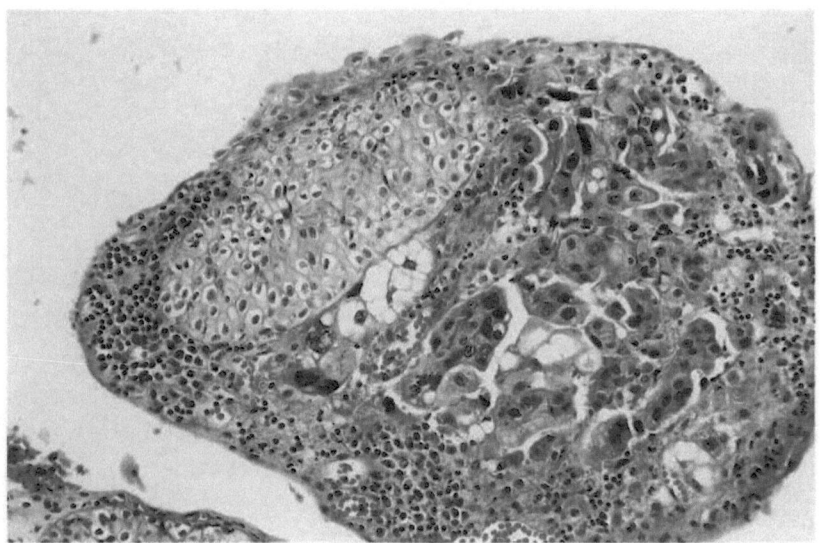

**Fig. 62.** *Urothelial carcinoma, micropapillary and lipid cell variants.* Both are present in this case of urothelial carcinoma

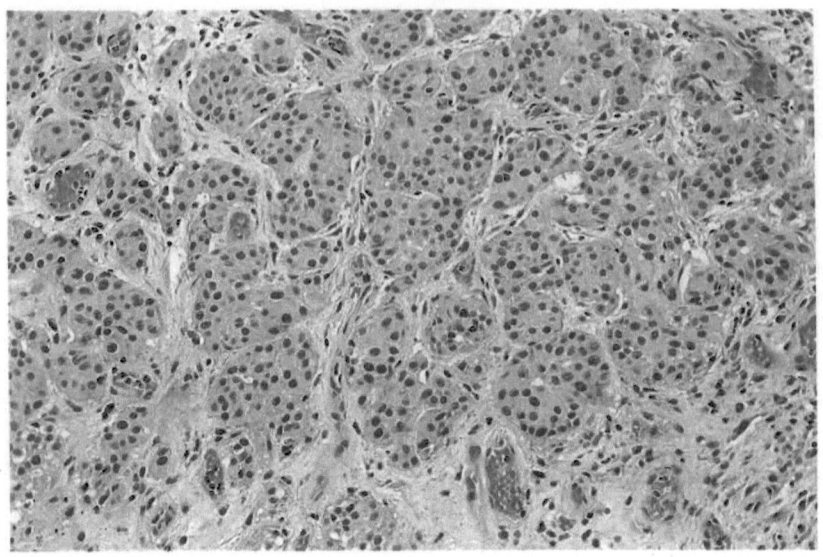

**Fig. 63.** *Urothelial carcinoma, nested variant*

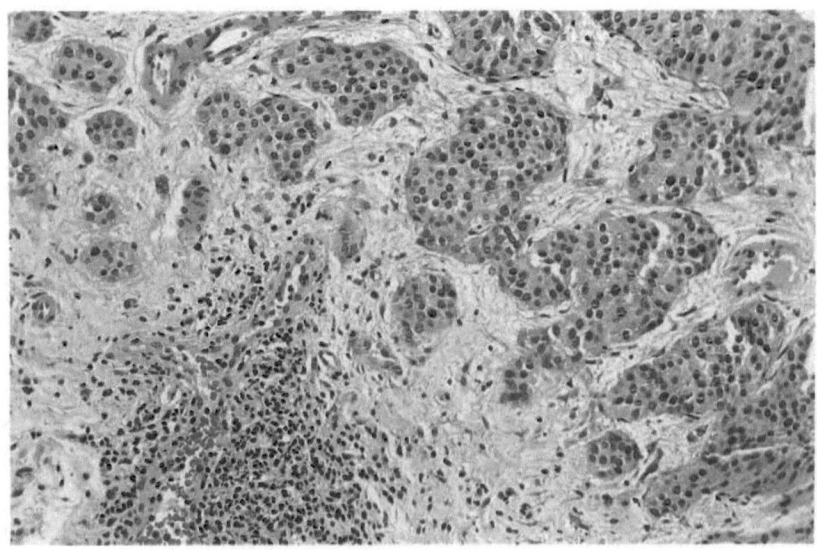

**Fig. 64.** *Urothelial carcinoma, nested variant*

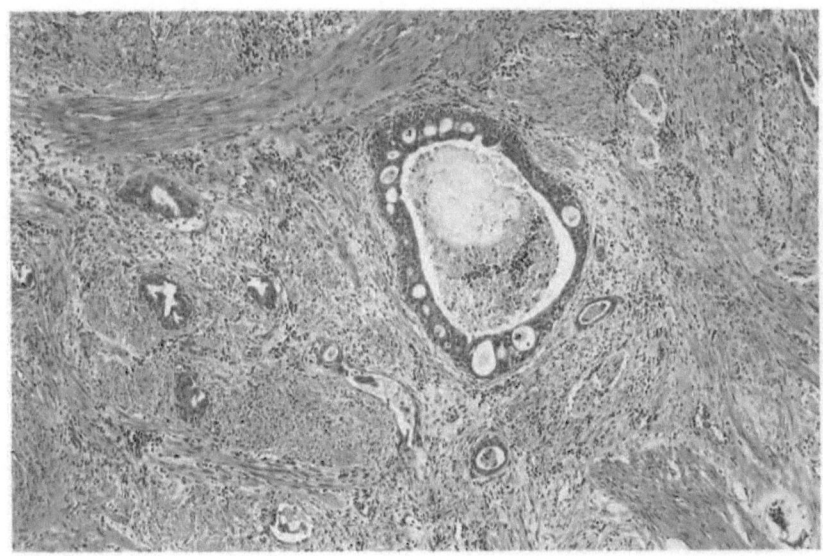

**Fig. 65.** *Urothelial carcinoma, microcystic variant.* Invasion of muscularis propria

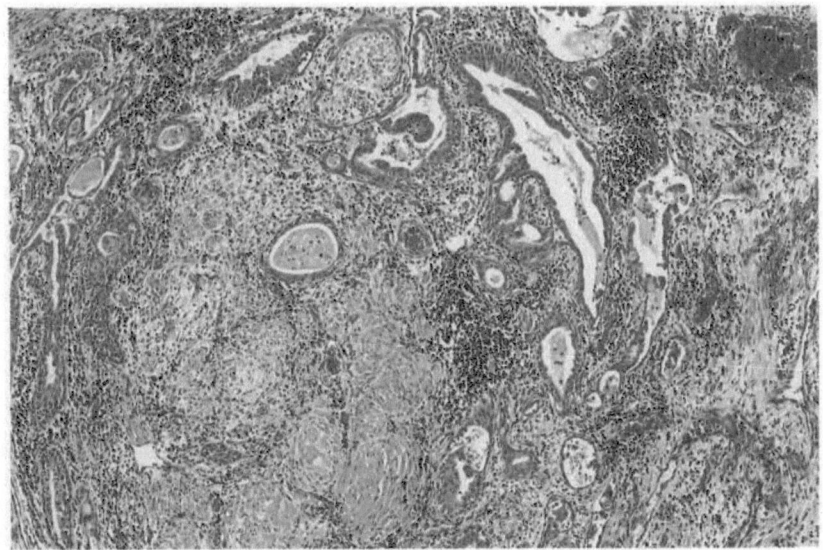

**Fig. 66.** *Urothelial carcinoma, microcystic variant*

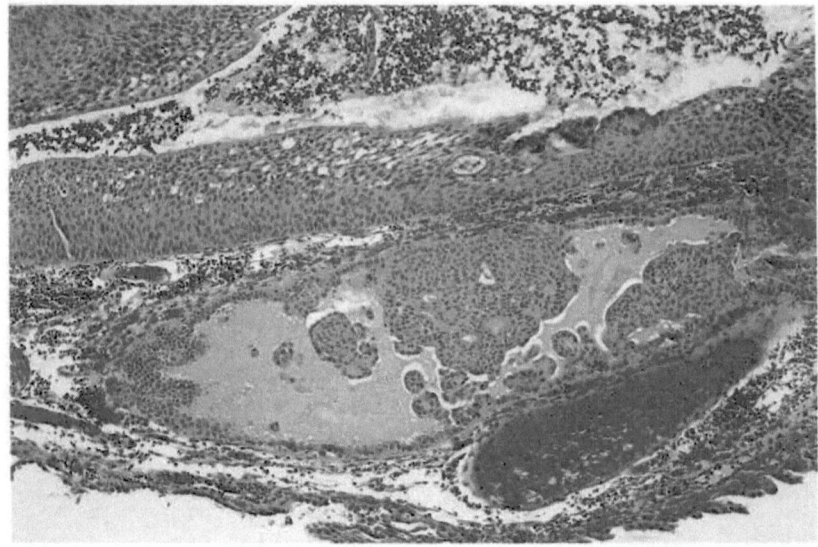

**Fig. 67.** *Urothelial carcinoma, microcystic variant.* Typical elements of urothelial carcinoma are also present

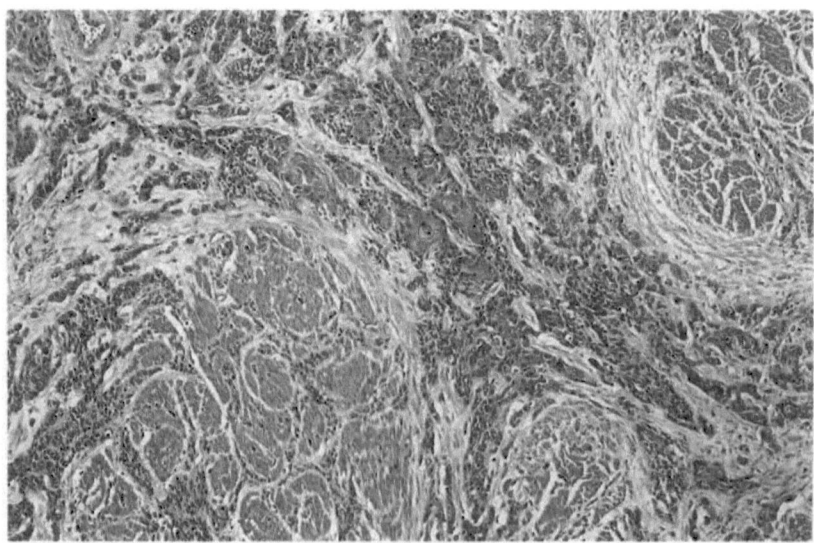

**Fig. 68.** *Squamous cell carcinoma* infiltrating muscularis propria

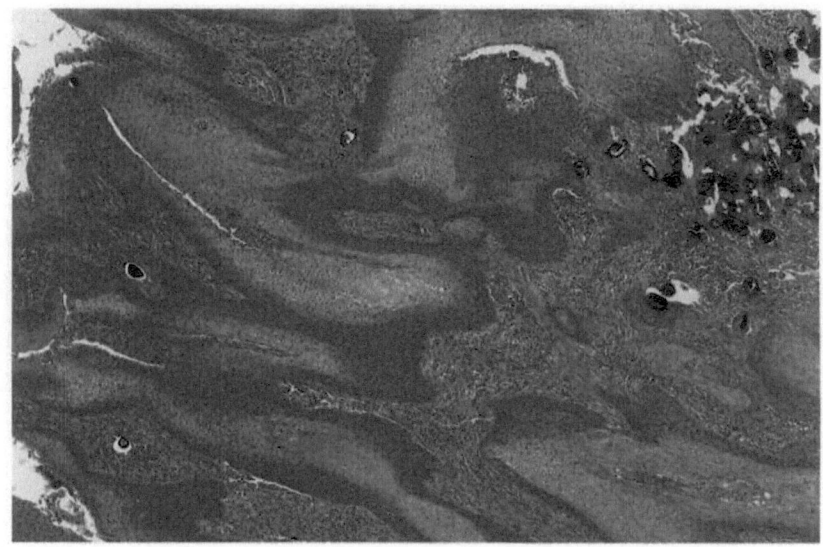

**Fig. 69.** *Squamous cell carcinoma* associated with schistosomiasis

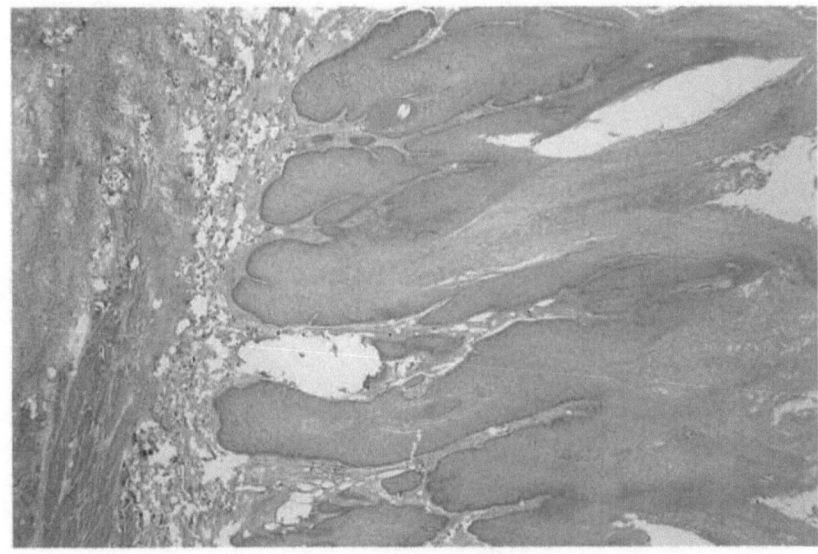

**Fig. 70.** *Verrucous carcinoma*

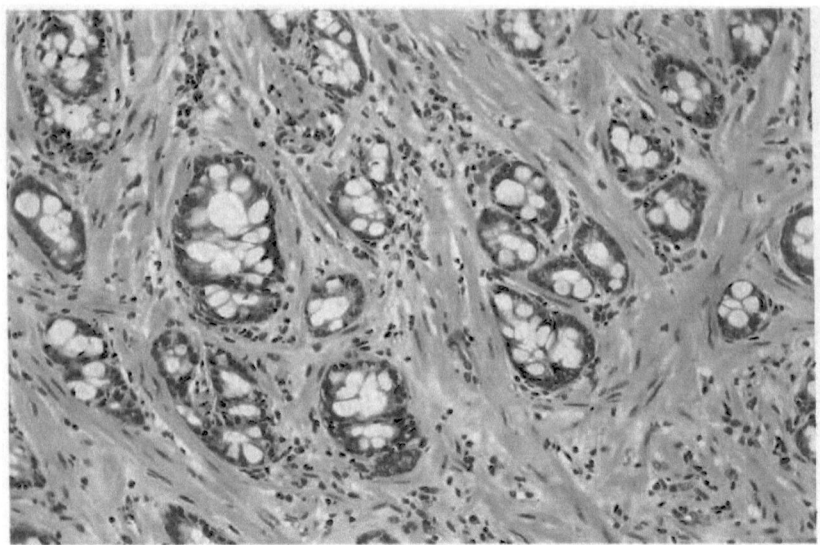

**Fig. 71.** *Adenocarcinoma, well differentiated*

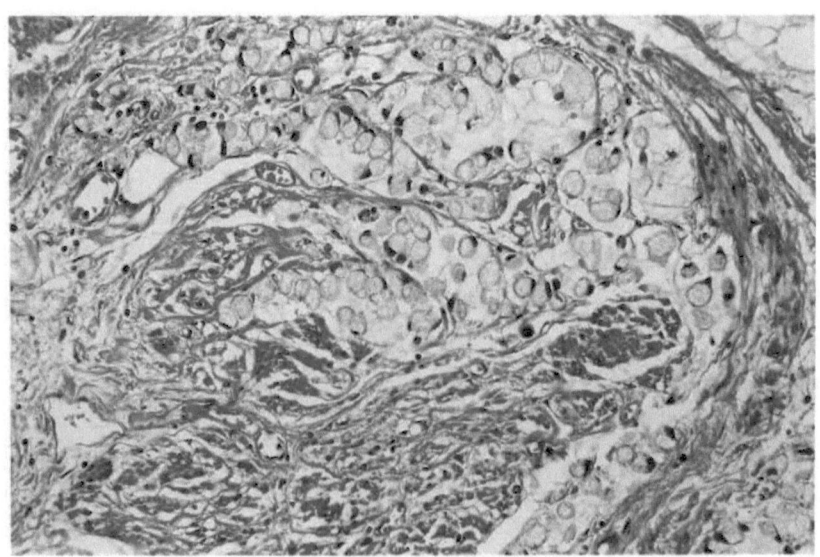

**Fig. 72.** *Signet-ring cell adenocarcinoma*

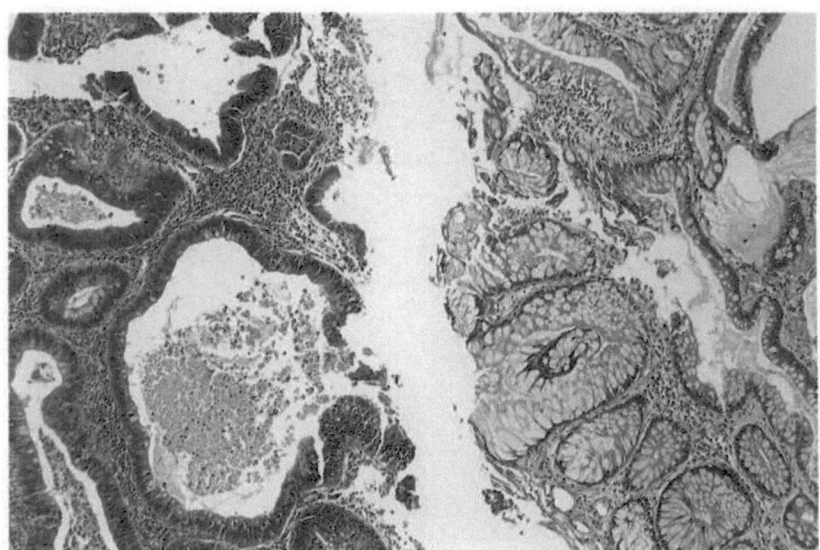

**Fig. 73.** *Adenocarcinoma* associated with cystitis glandularis

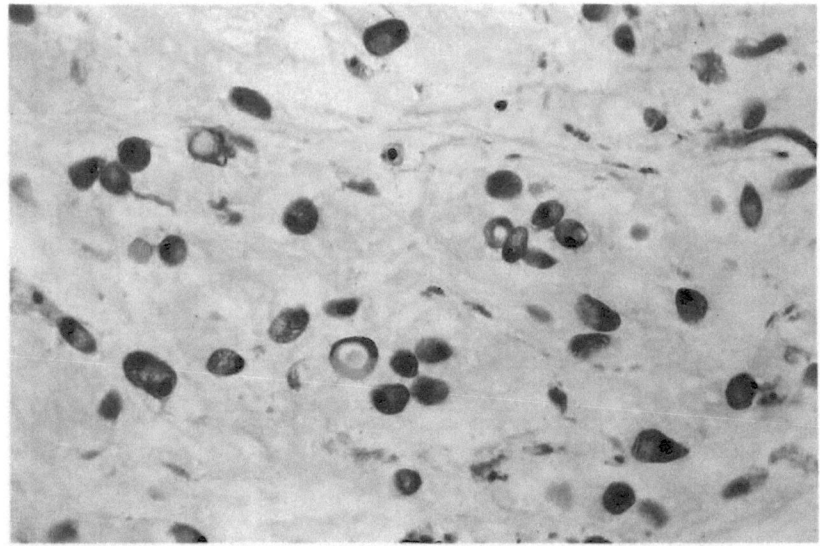

**Fig. 74.** *Signet-ring cell adenocarcinoma.* This field also shows plasmacytoid features

70

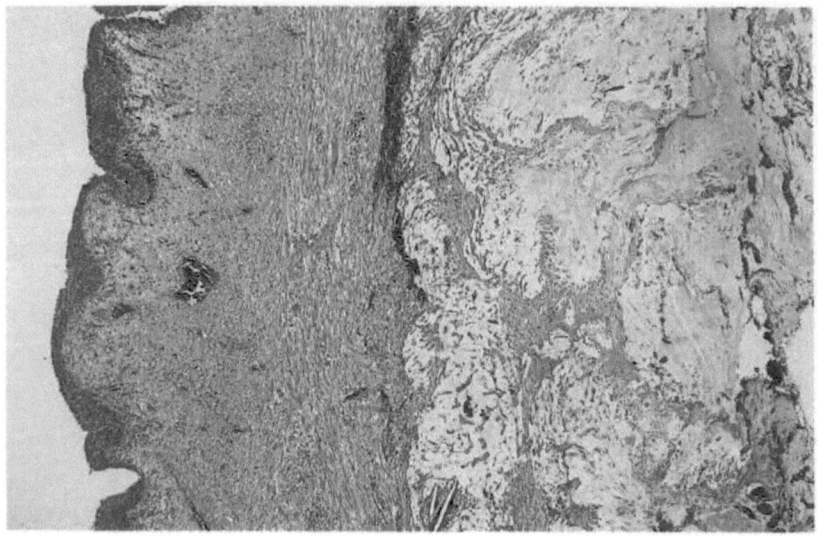

**Fig. 75.** *Urachal carcinoma.* The bladder mucosa (*left*) is normal and the mucinous carcinoma occupies the muscularis propria

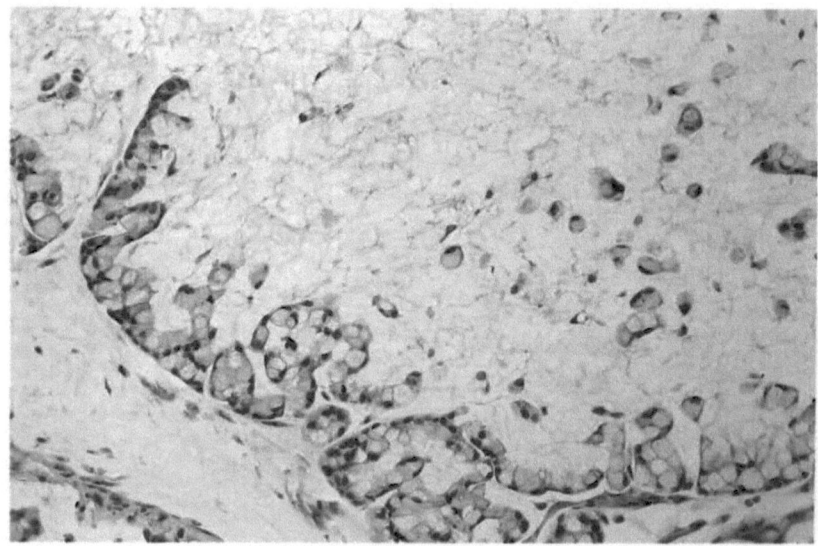

**Fig. 76.** *Urachal carcinoma*

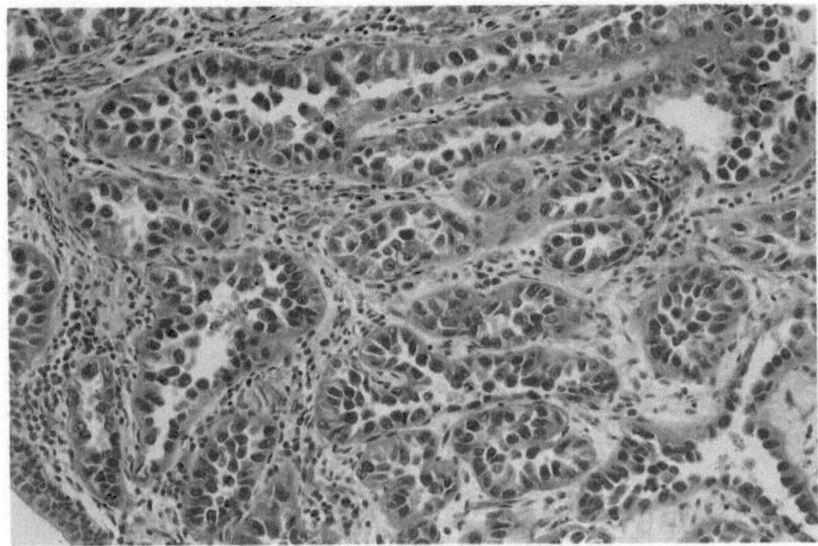

**Fig. 77.** *Clear cell adenocarcinoma.* Although clear cells are often not prominent, tubular morphology and hobnail features are typical

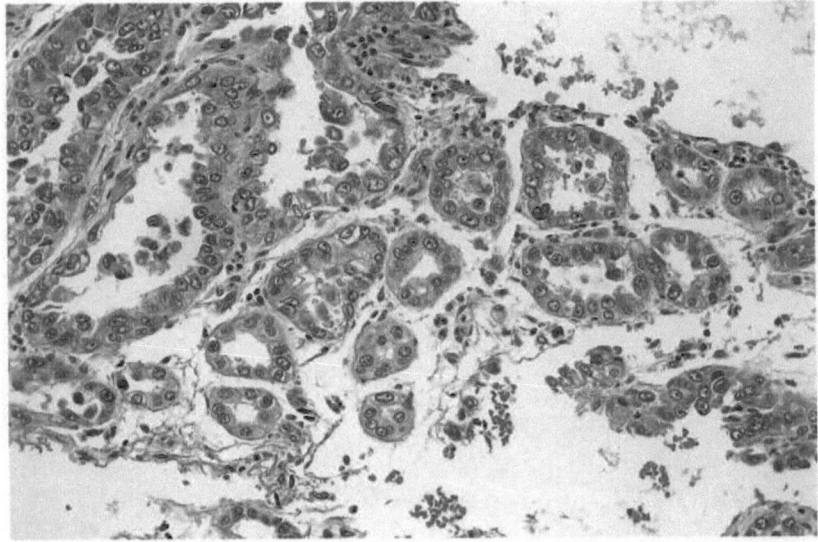

**Fig. 78.** *Clear cell adenocarcinoma.* Nuclear anaplasia distinguishes this from nephrogenic adenoma

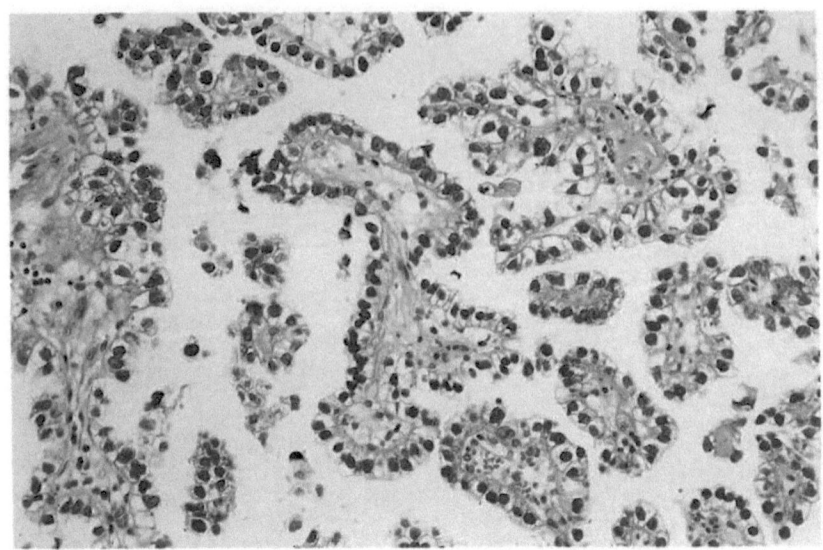

**Fig. 79.** *Clear cell adenocarcinoma.* Papillary pattern with clear cells

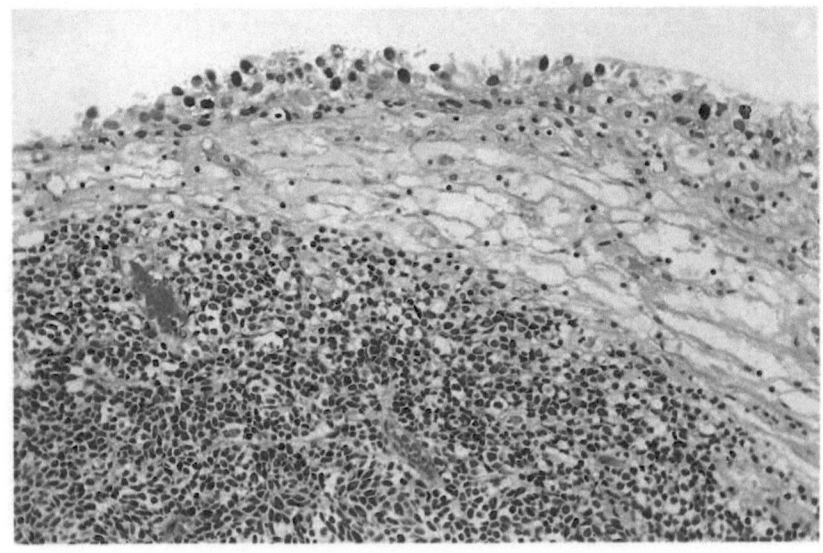

**Fig. 80.** *Small cell carcinoma.* Urothelial carcinoma in situ is also present

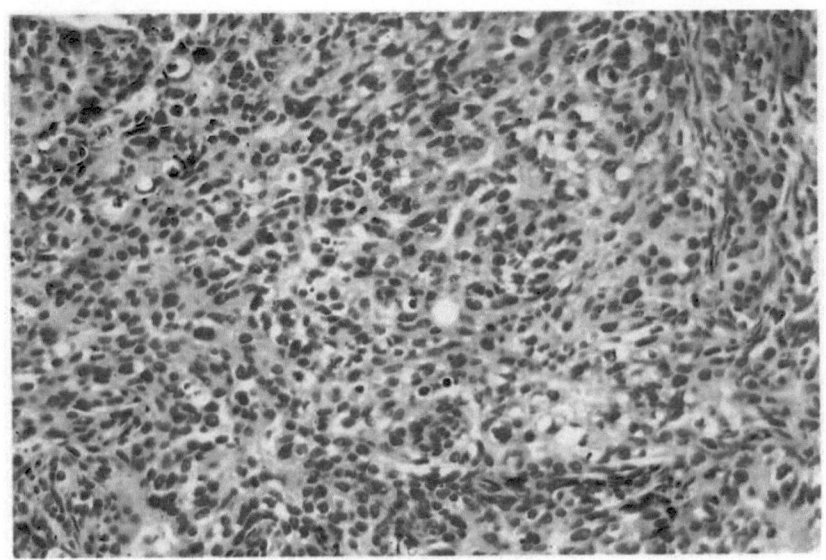

**Fig. 81.** *Undifferentiated carcinoma*

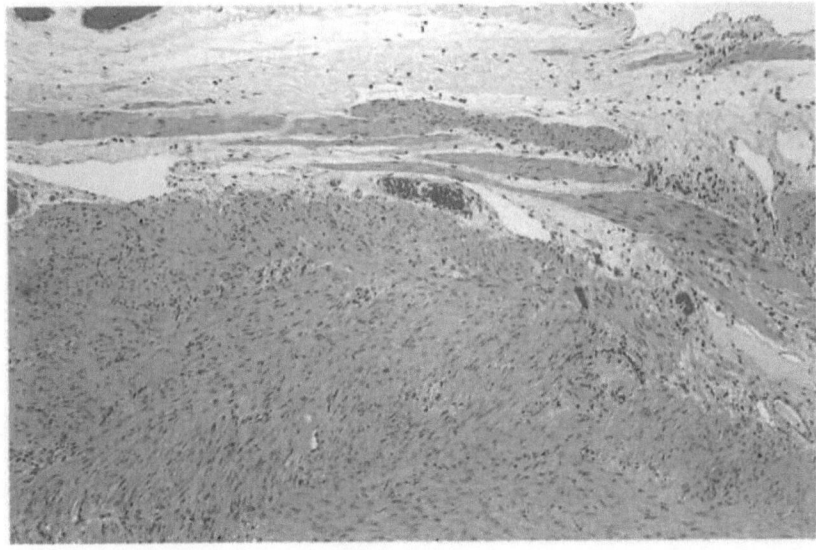

**Fig. 82.** *Leiomyoma*

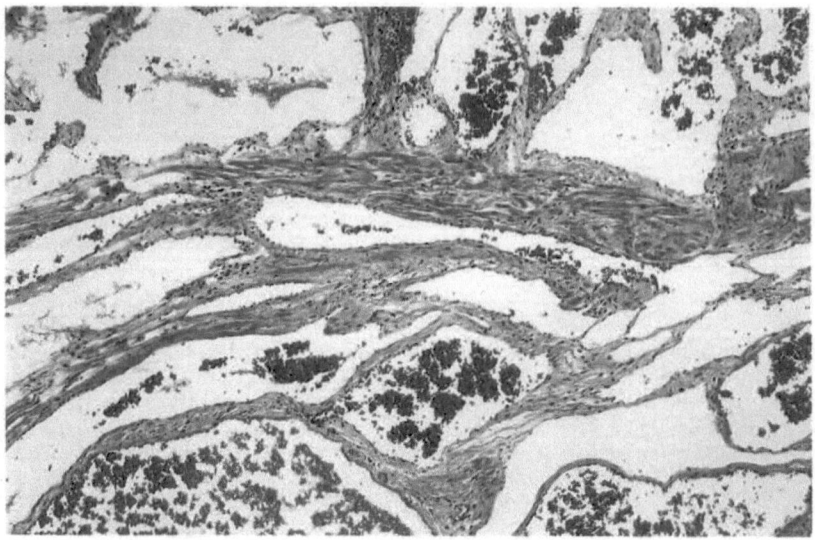

**Fig. 83.** *Haemangioma*

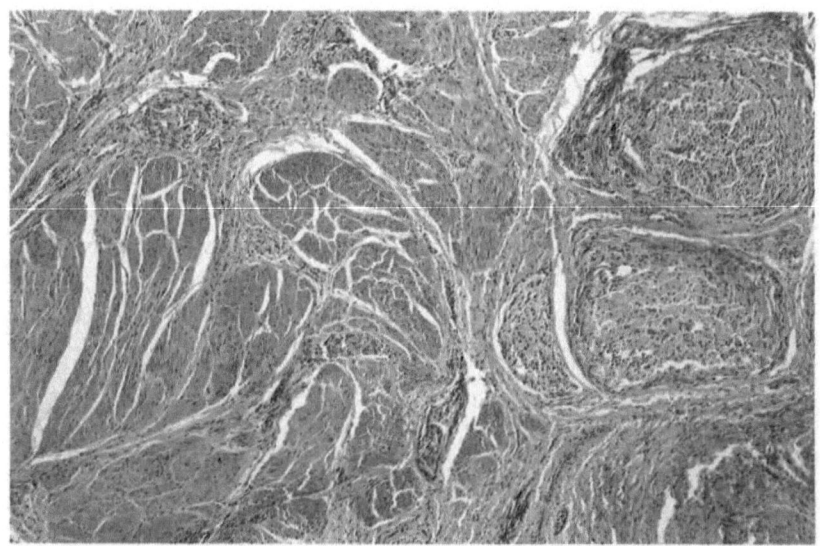

**Fig. 84.** *Neurofibroma*

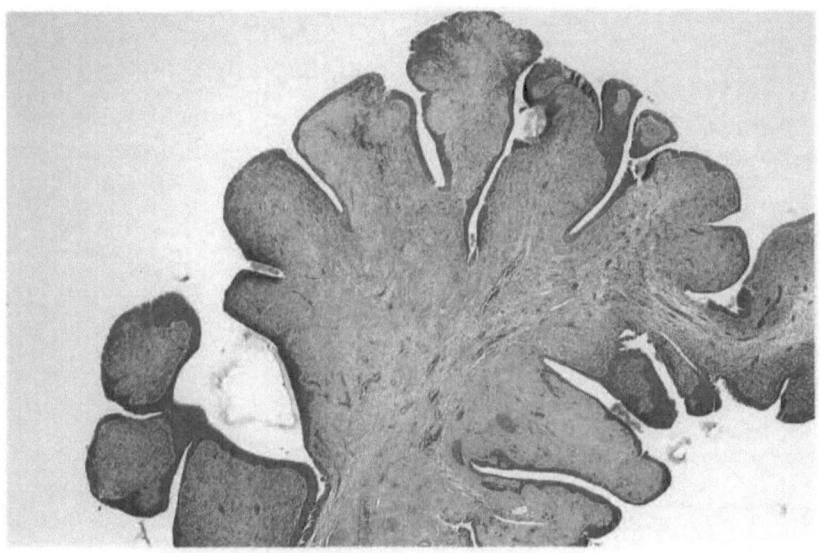

**Fig. 85.** *Rhabdomyosarcoma (sarcoma botryoides)*

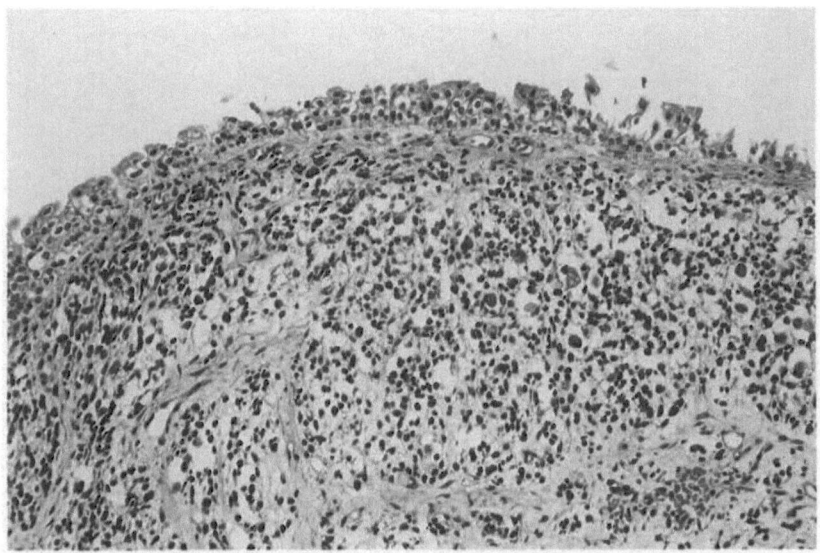

**Fig. 86.** *Embryonal rhabdomyosarcoma.* Dense cambian layer of sarcoma botryoides

76

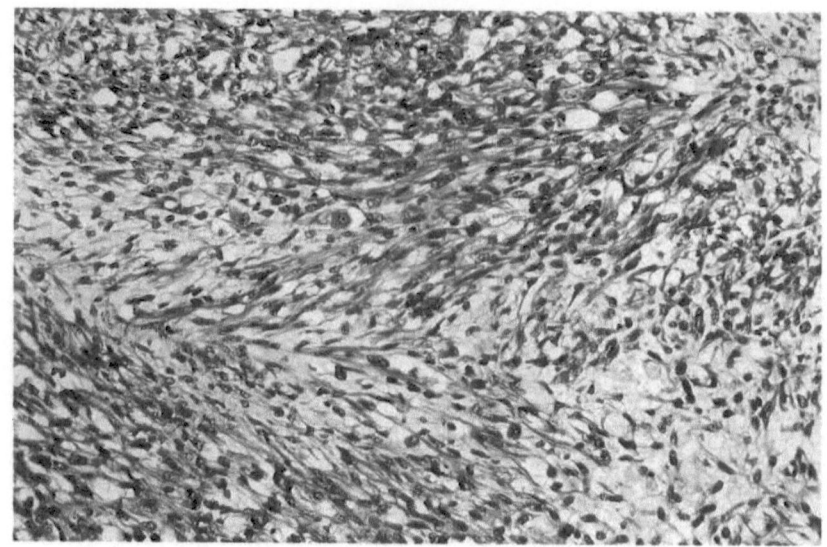

**Fig. 87.** *Embryonal rhabdomyosarcoma*

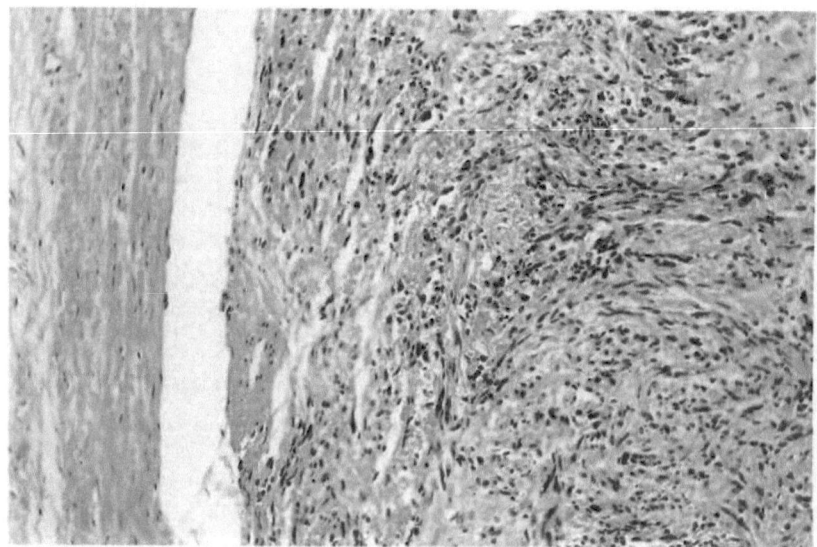

**Fig. 88.** *Leiomyosarcoma*

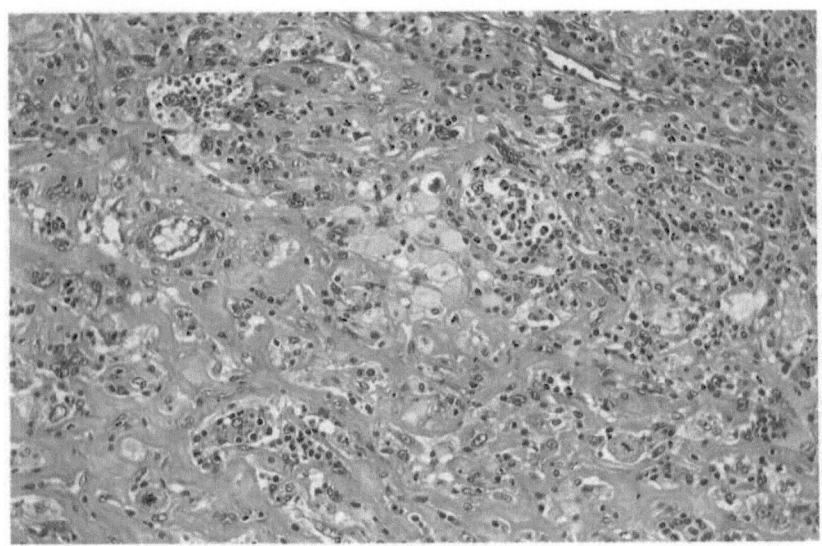

**Fig. 89.** *Malignant fibrous histiocytoma*

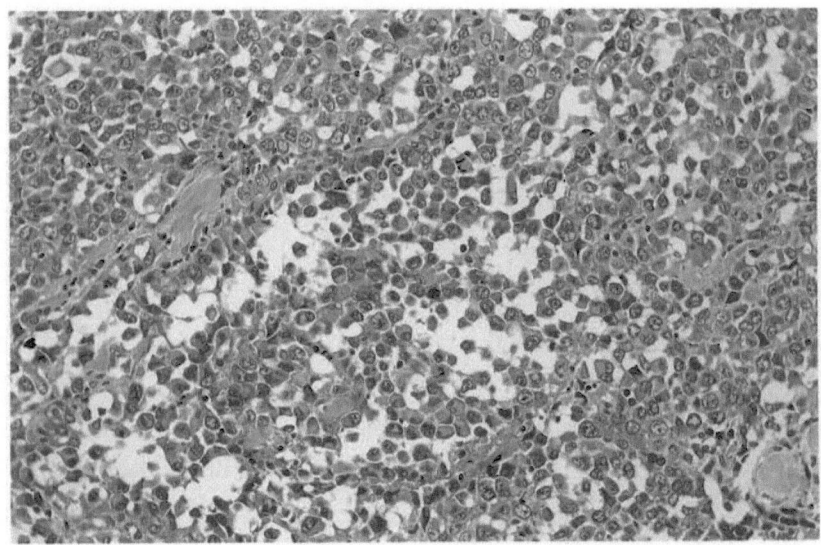

**Fig. 90.** *Malignant rhabdoid tumour*

78

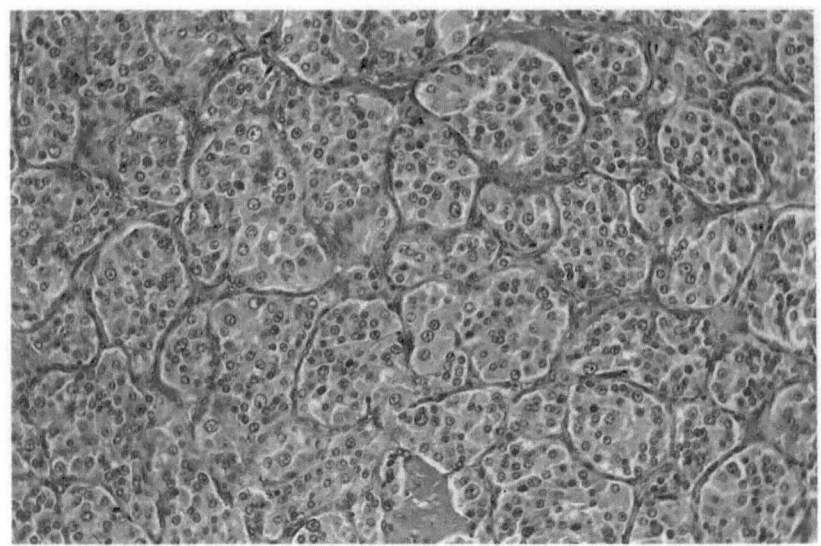

**Fig. 91.** *Paraganglioma*

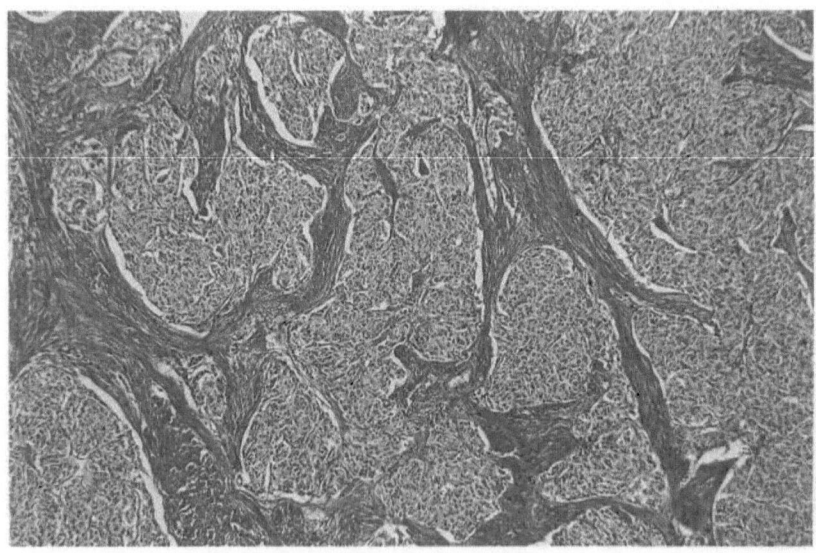

**Fig. 92.** *Paraganglioma*

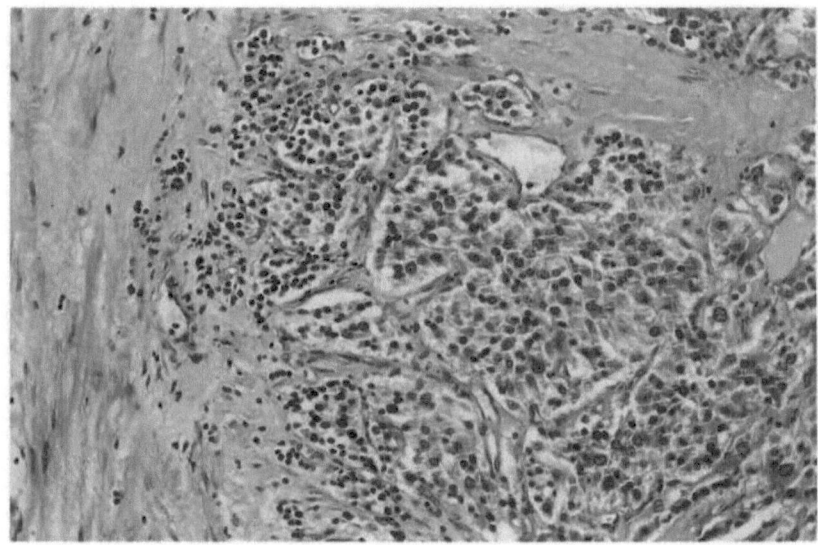

**Fig. 93.** *Paraganglioma.* Small, dark neuroblastoma-like cells are present near the bladder mucosa (*left*)

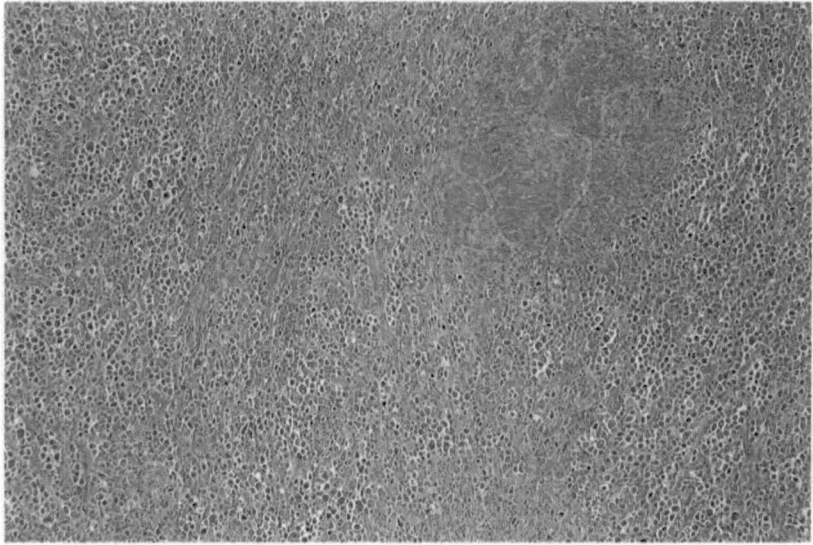

**Fig. 94.** *Malignant lymphoma.* Infiltrating muscularis propria

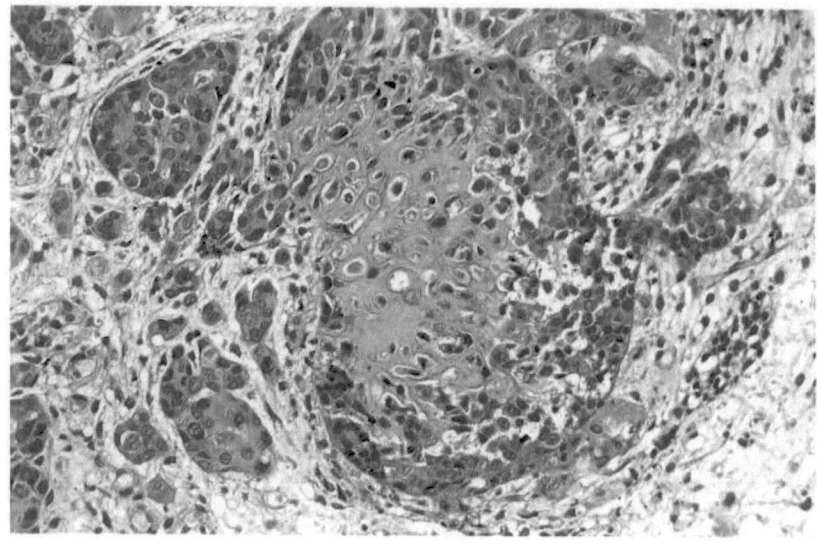

**Fig. 95.** *Carcinosarcoma.* Urothelial carcinoma and chondrosarcoma

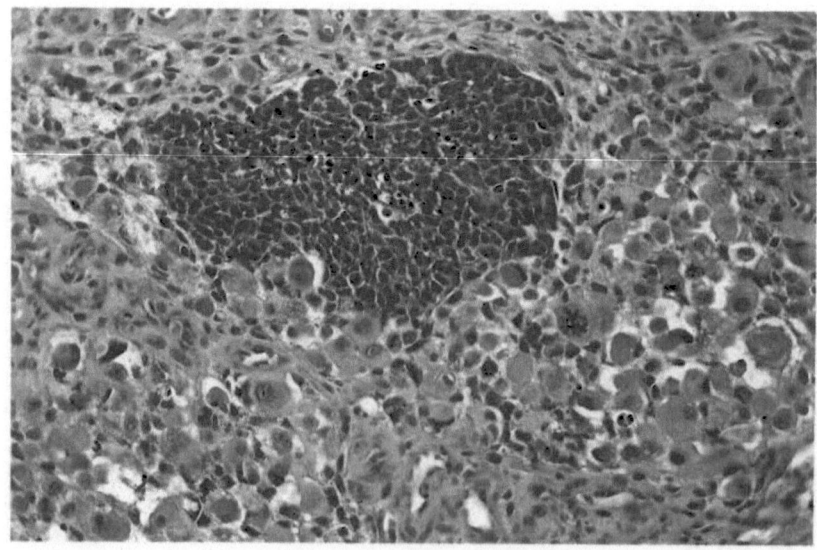

**Fig. 96.** *Carcinosarcoma.* Urothelial carcinoma and rhabdomyosarcoma

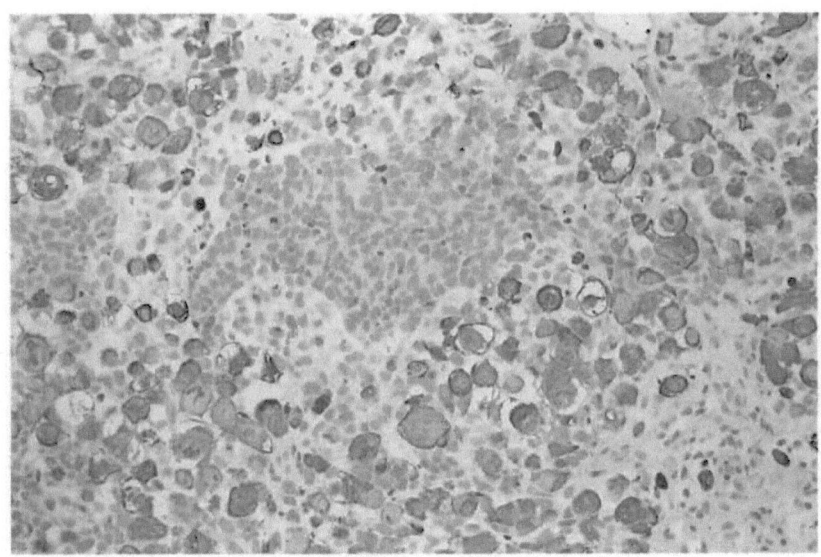

**Fig. 97.** *Carcinosarcoma.* Desmin reaction, same field as Fig. 96

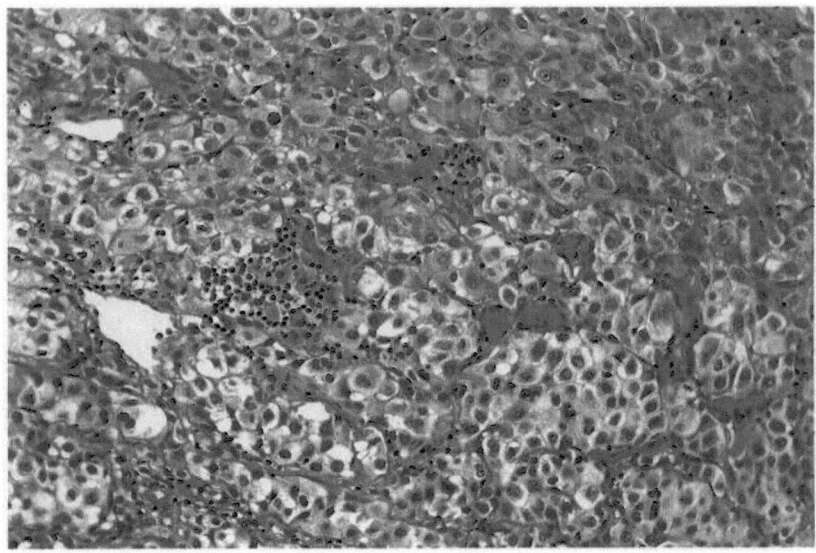

**Fig. 98.** *Malignant melanoma*

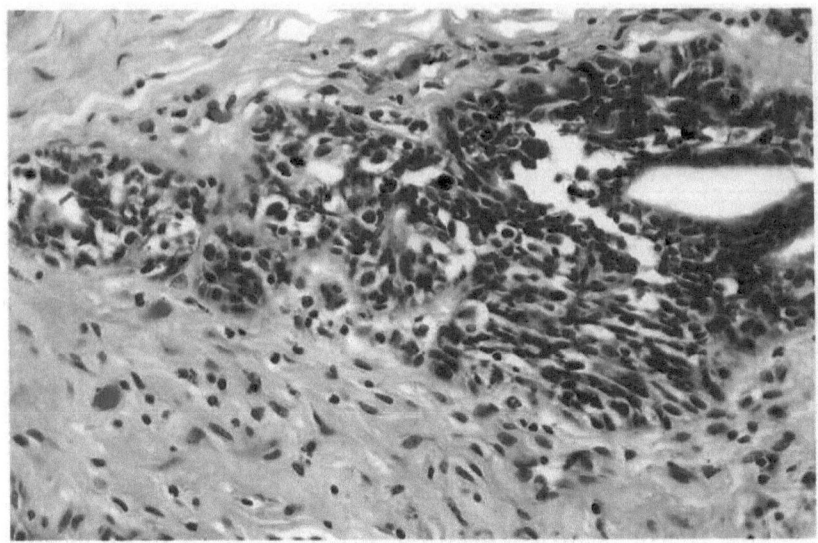

**Fig. 99.** *Atypical melanocytes.* A case of bladder melanoma

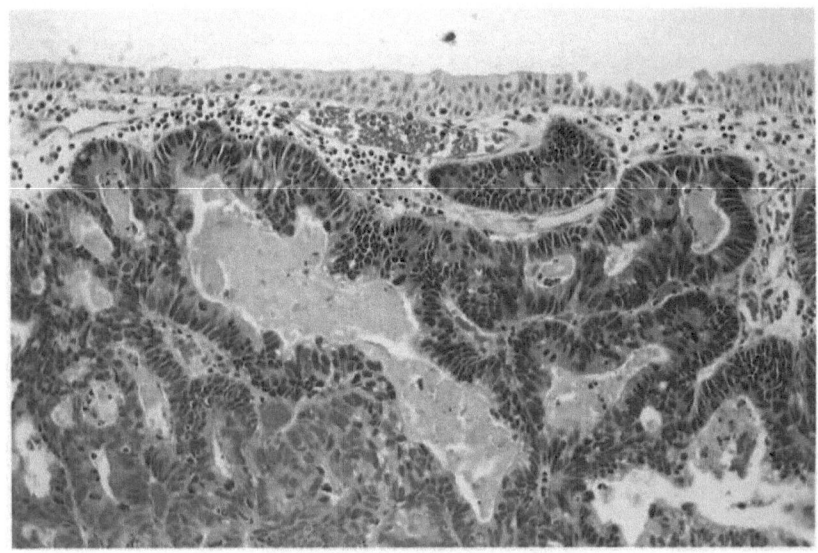

**Fig. 100.** Colonic adenocarcinoma invading through bladder wall. Note normal bladder epithelium

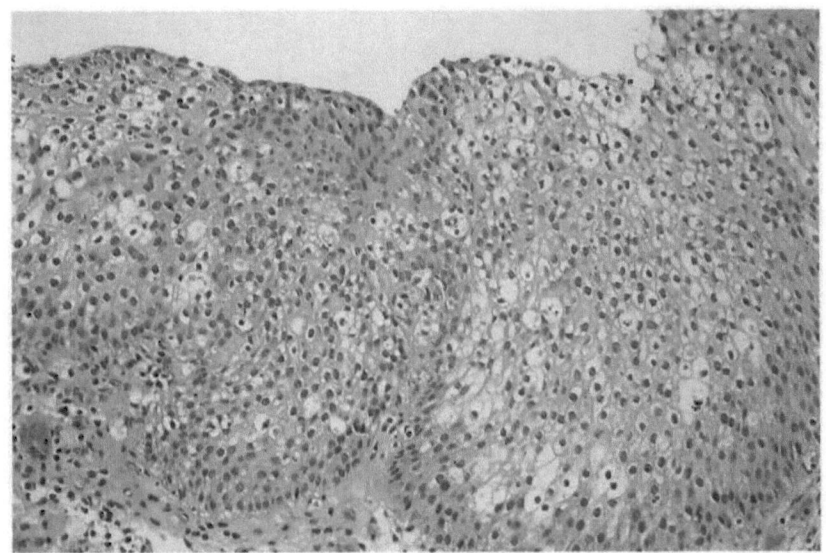

**Fig. 101.** *Flat urothelial hyperplasia*

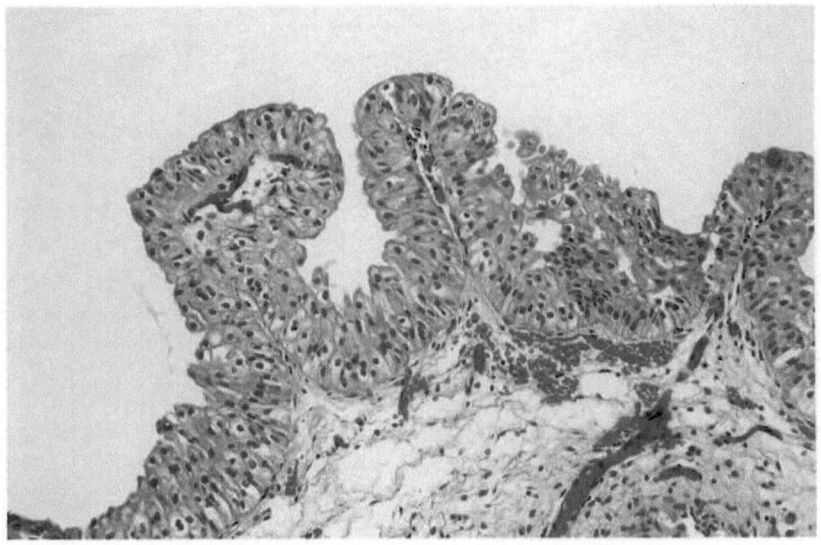

**Fig. 102.** *Papillary urothelial hyperplasia*

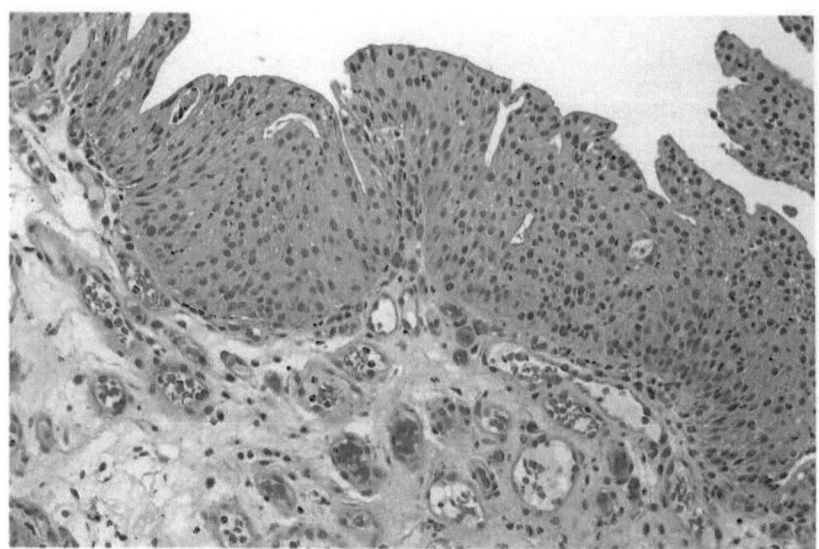

**Fig. 103.** *Reactive atypia*

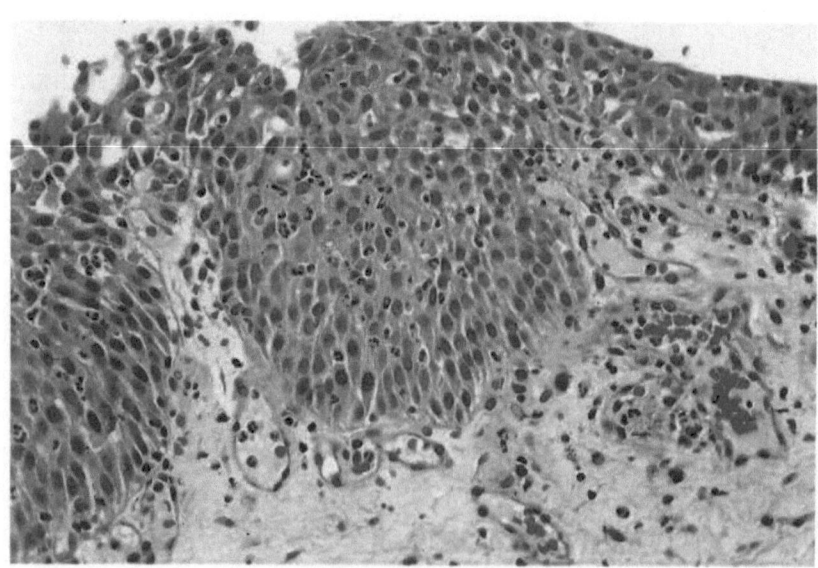

**Fig. 104.** *Reactive atypia*

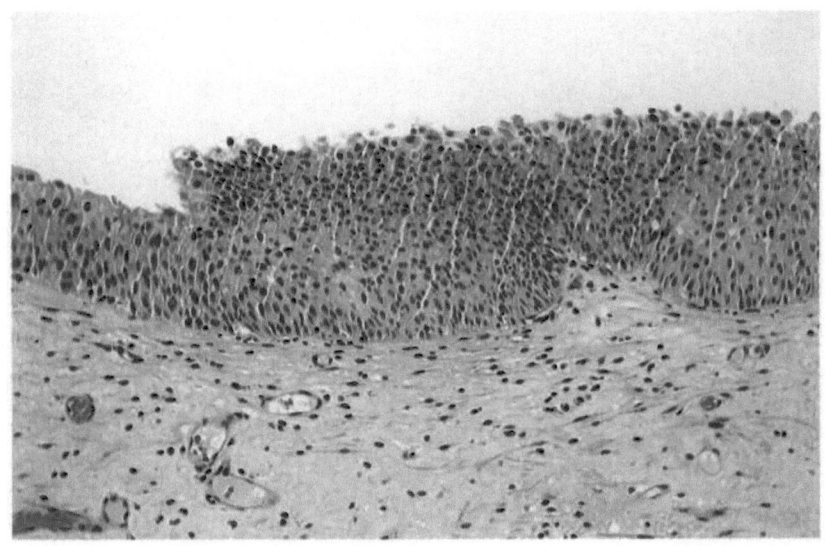

**Fig. 105.** *Atypia of uncertain significance*

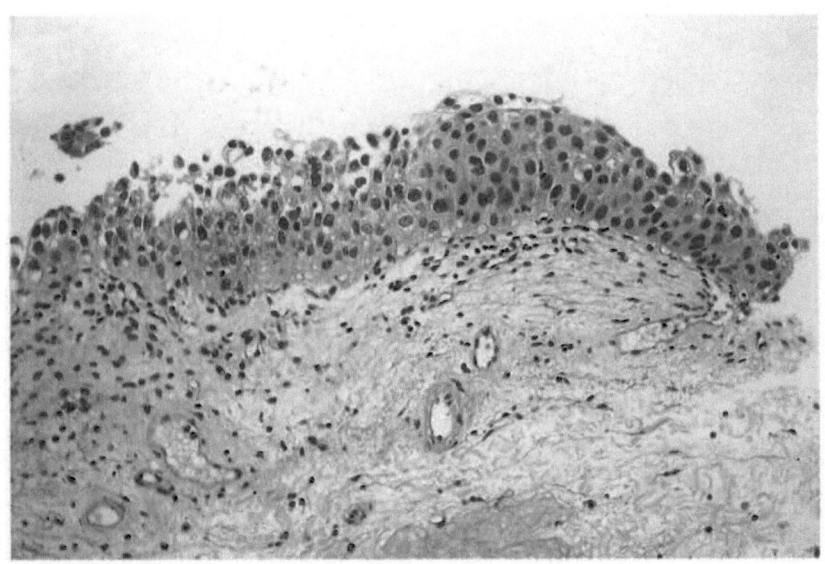

**Fig. 106.** *Atypia of uncertain significance*

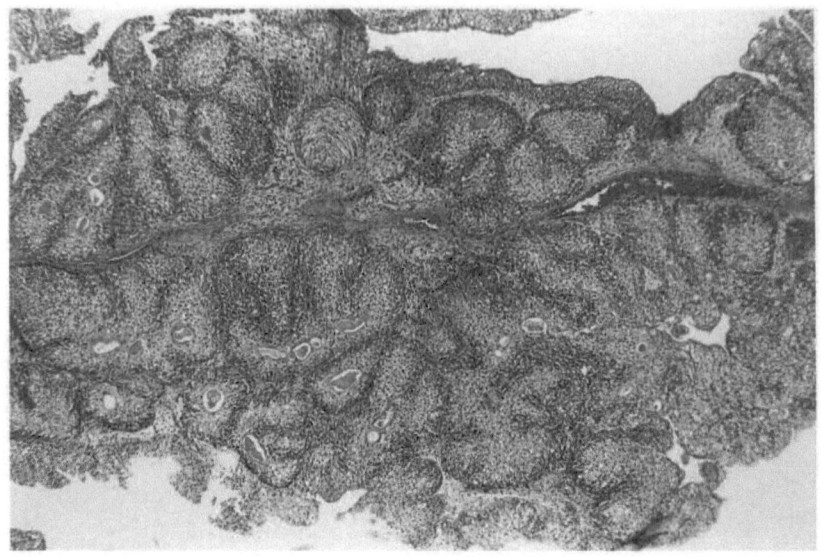

**Fig. 107.** *Von Brunn nests*

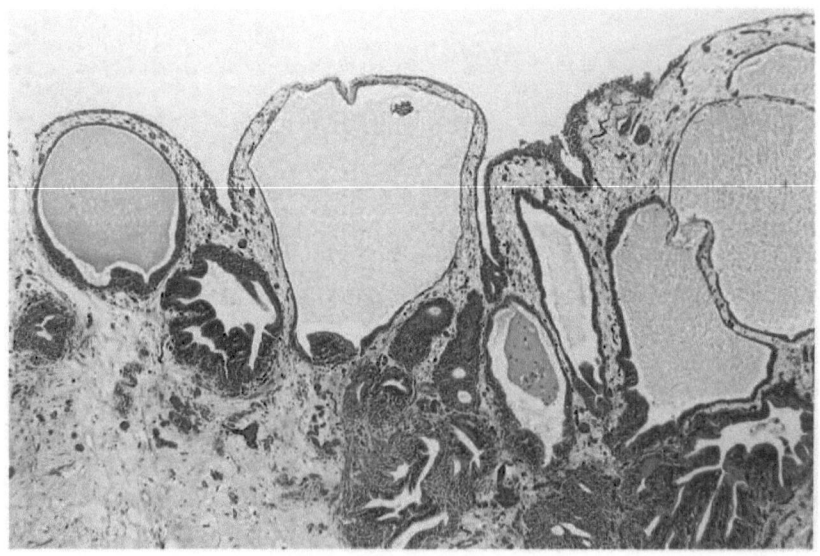

**Fig. 108.** *Cystitis cystica*

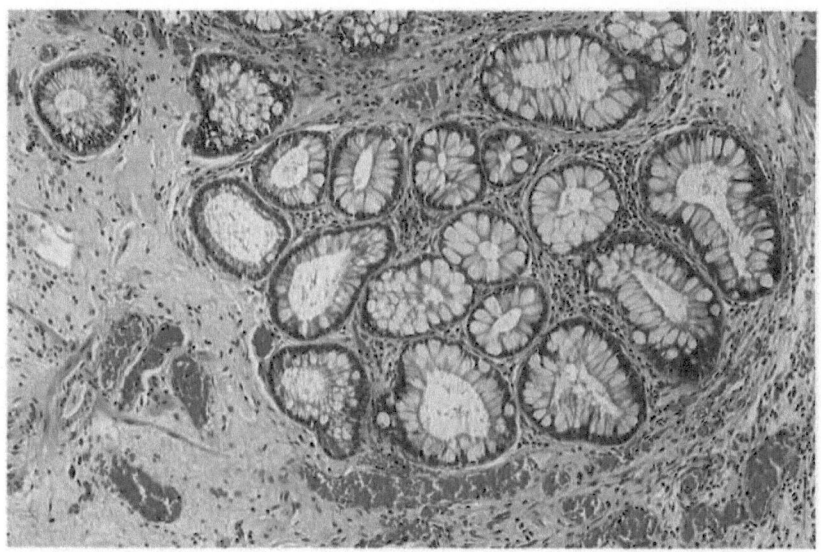

**Fig. 109.** *Cystitis glandularis*

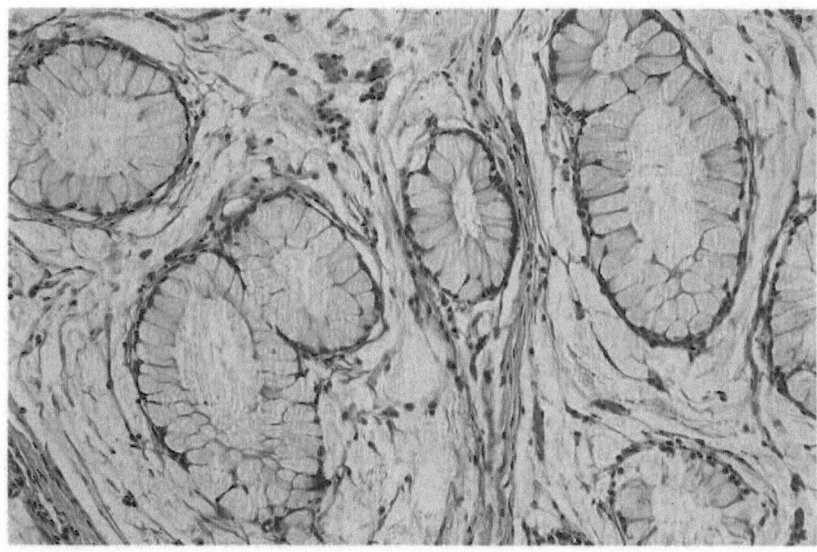

**Fig. 110.** *Cystitis glandularis*. Extravasated lakes of mucin

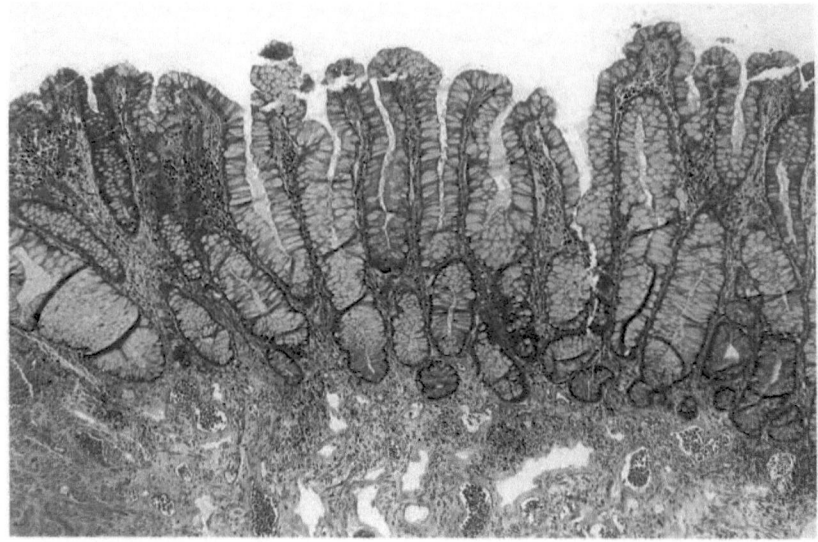

**Fig. 111.** *Intestinal metaplasia*

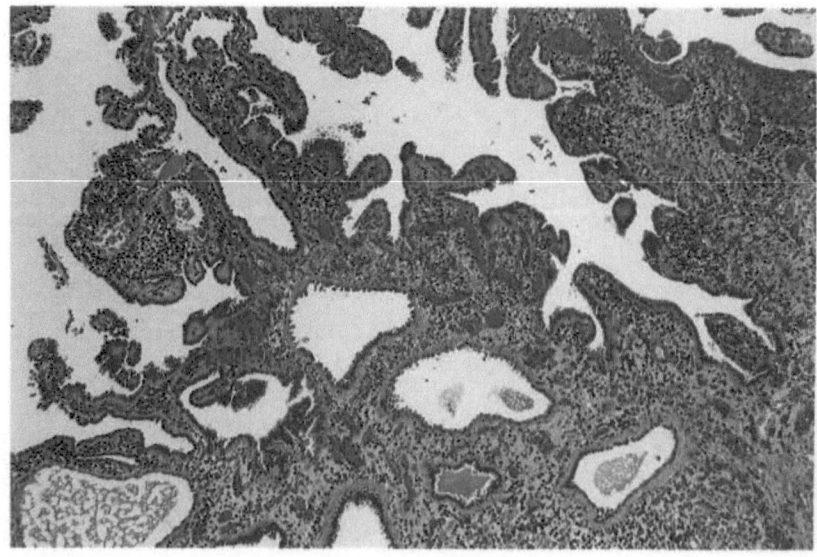

**Fig. 112.** *Nephrogenic adenoma*

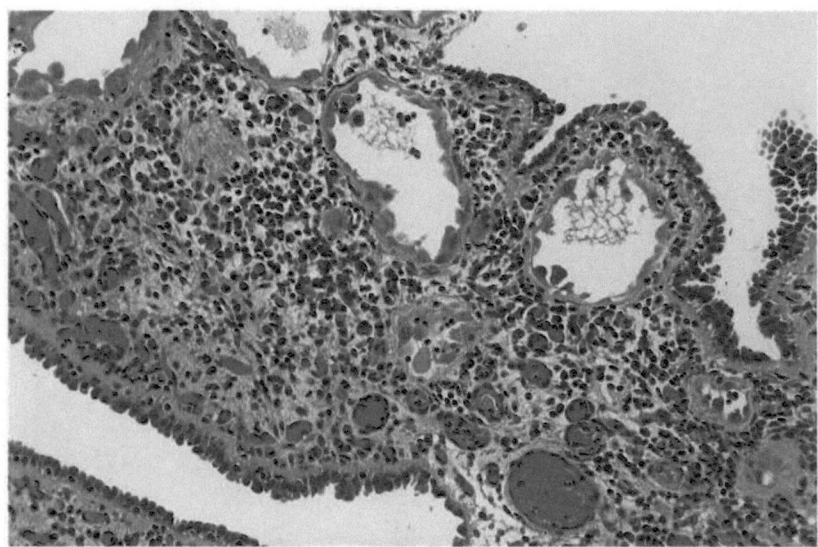

**Fig. 113.** *Nephrogenic adenoma*

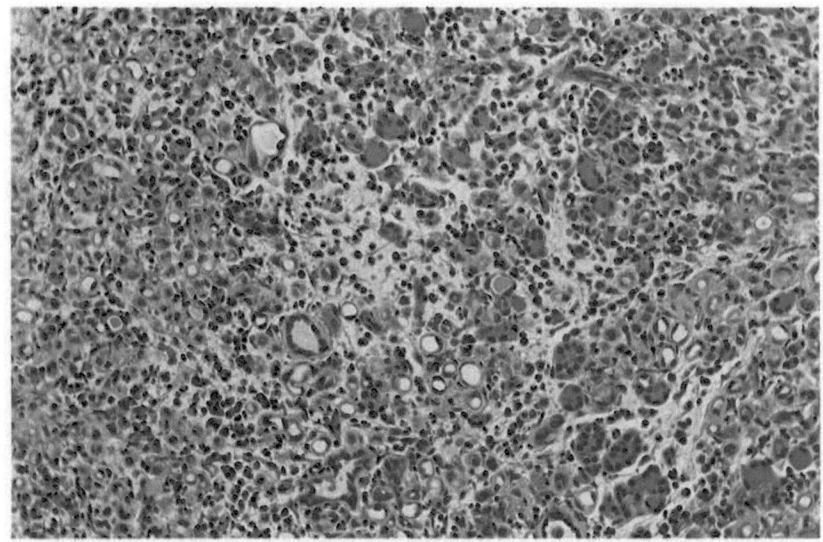

**Fig. 114.** *Nephrogenic adenoma*

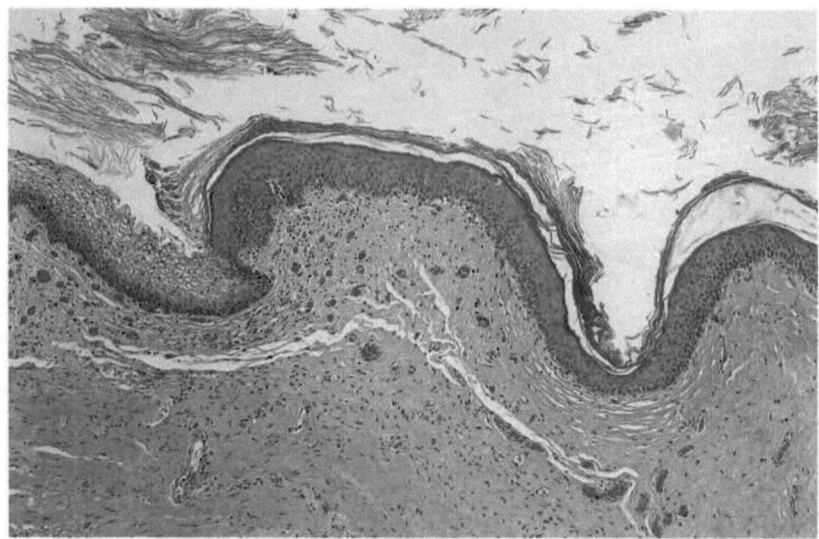

**Fig. 115.** *Keratinizing squamous metaplasia.* Non-keratinizing trigonal-type epithelium at the *left*

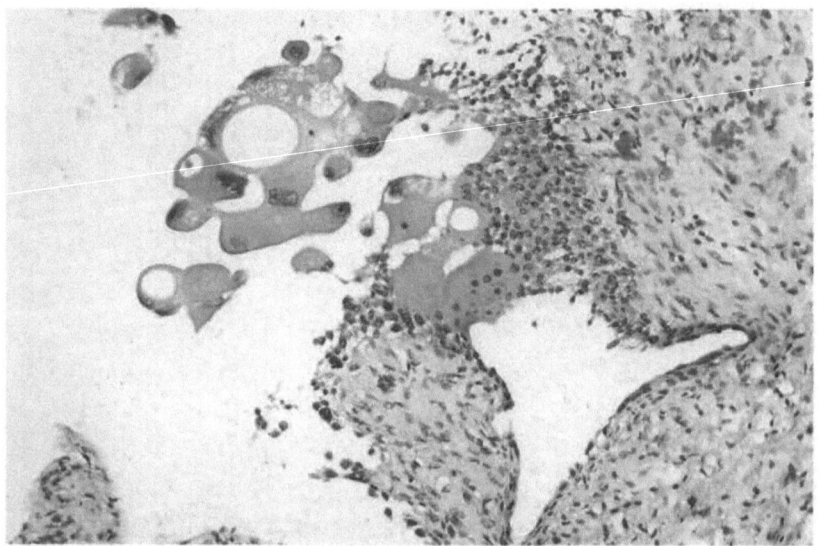

**Fig. 116.** *Thiotepa effect*

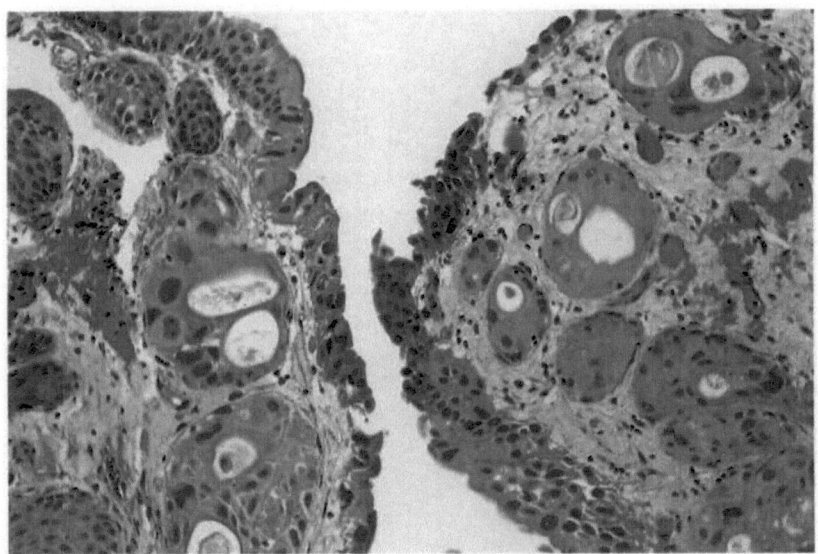

**Fig. 117.** *Thiotepa effect*

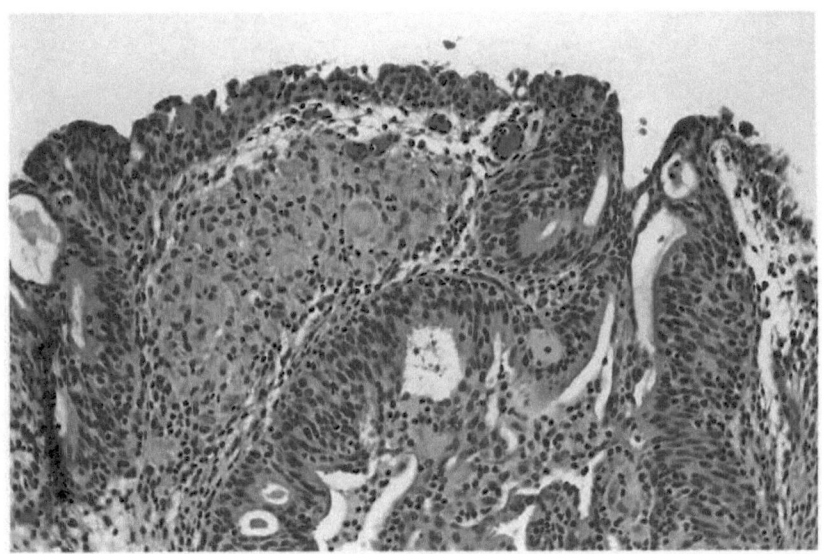

**Fig. 118.** *Granuloma due to bacillus Calmette-Guérin therapy*

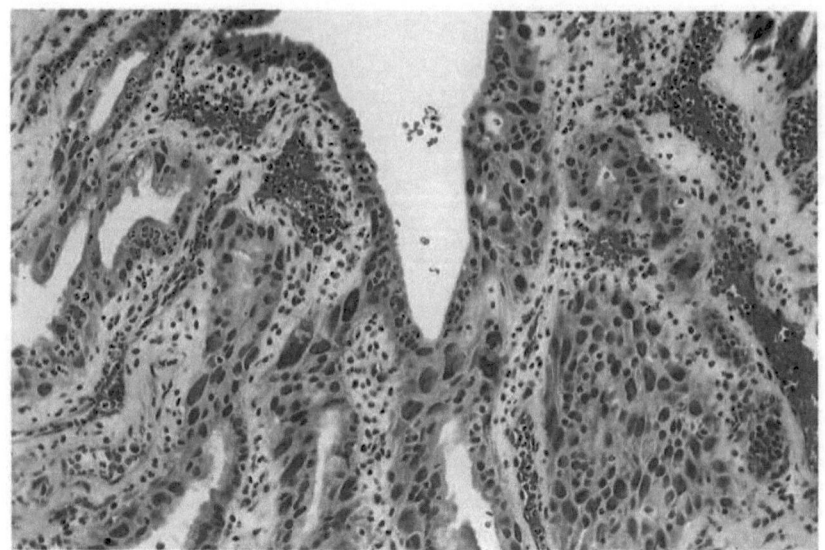

**Fig. 119.** *Radiation effect*

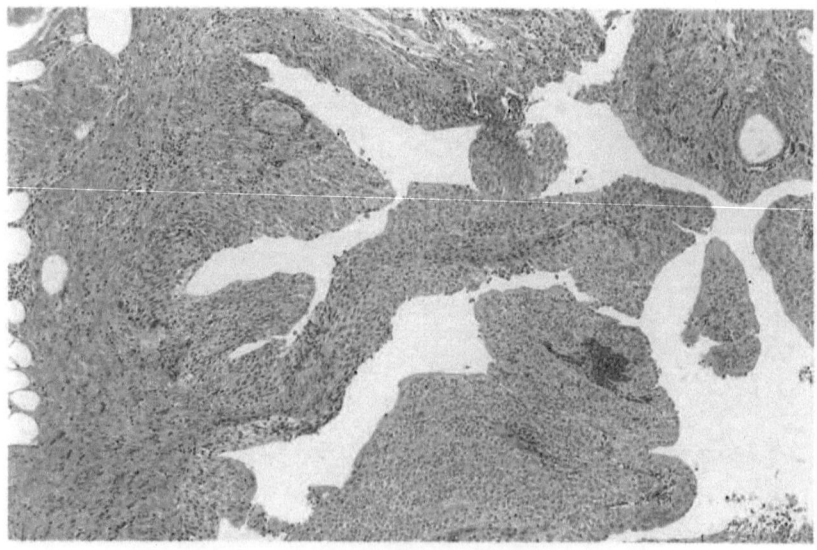

**Fig. 120.** *Papillary cystitis*. Site of a colovesical fistula

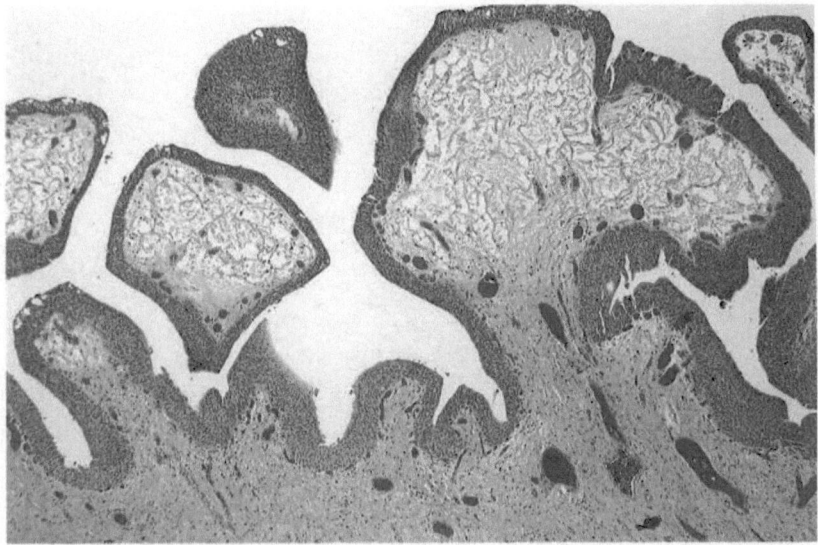

**Fig. 121.** *Polypoid cystitis*

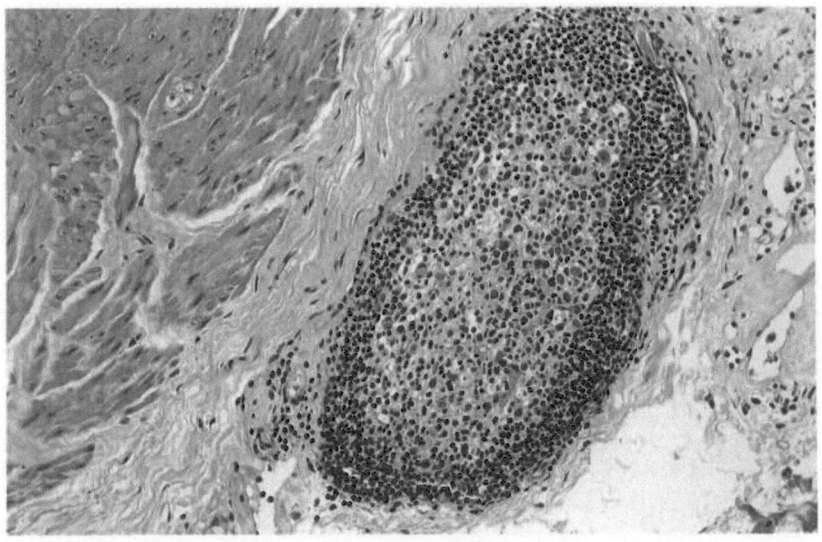

**Fig. 122.** *Follicular cystitis*

94

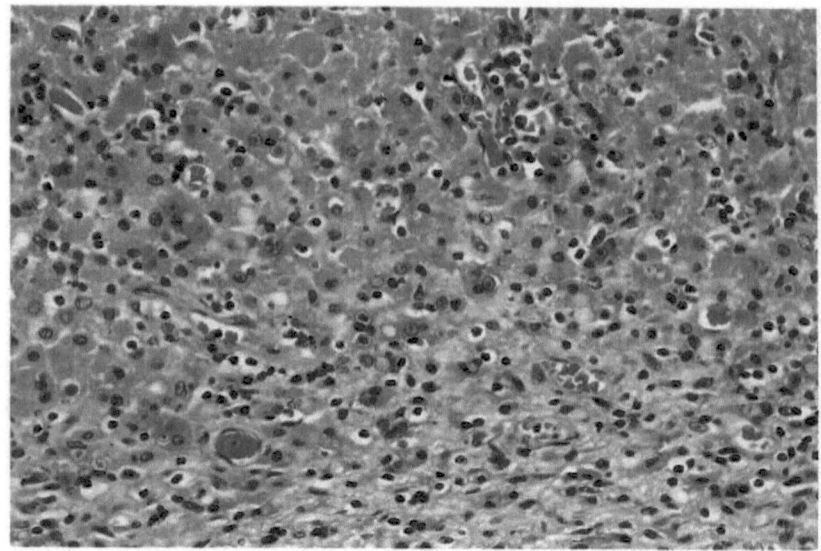

**Fig. 123.** *Malakoplakia*

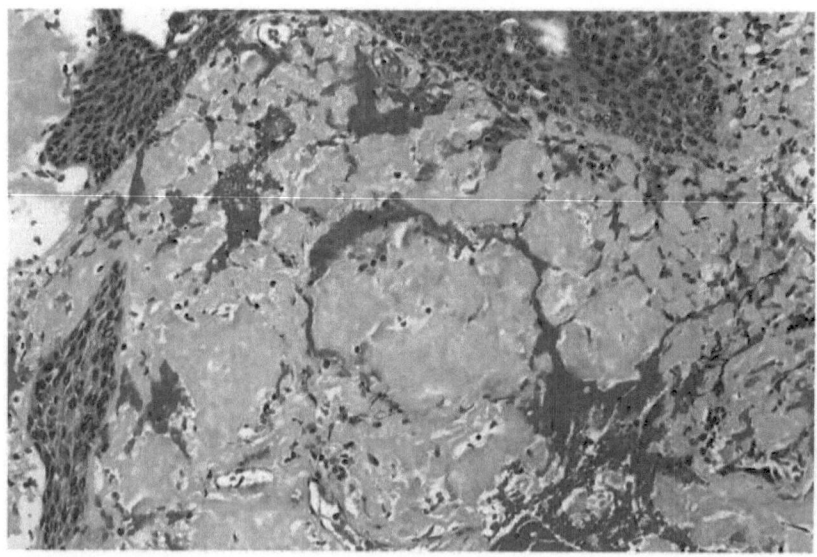

**Fig. 124.** *Amyloidosis*

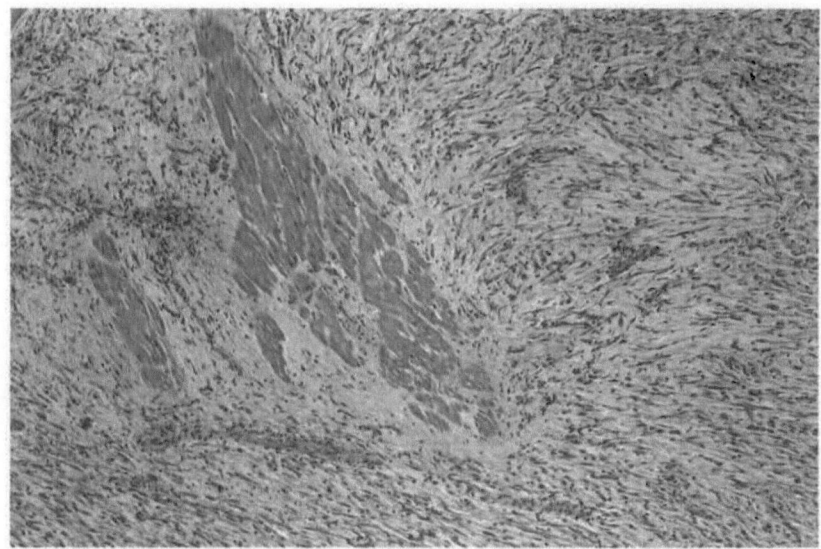

**Fig. 125.** *Myofibroblastic tumour* in muscularis propria

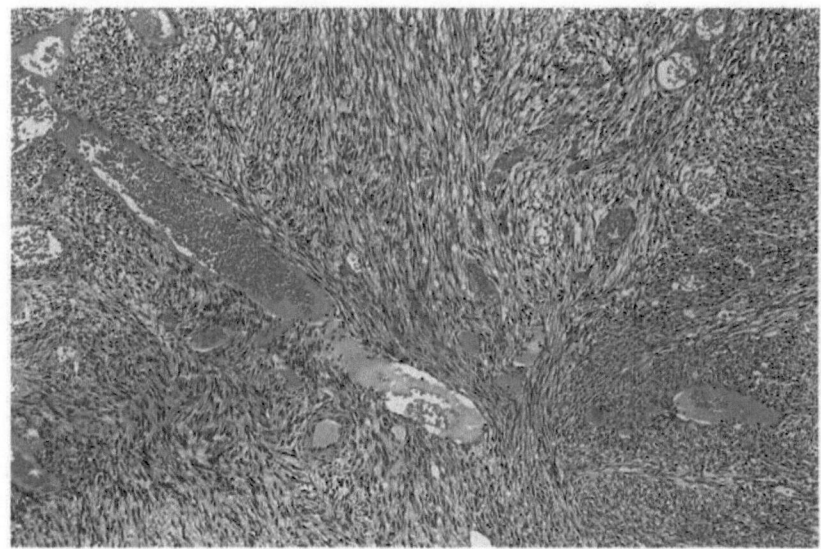

**Fig. 126.** *Postoperative spindle cell nodule*

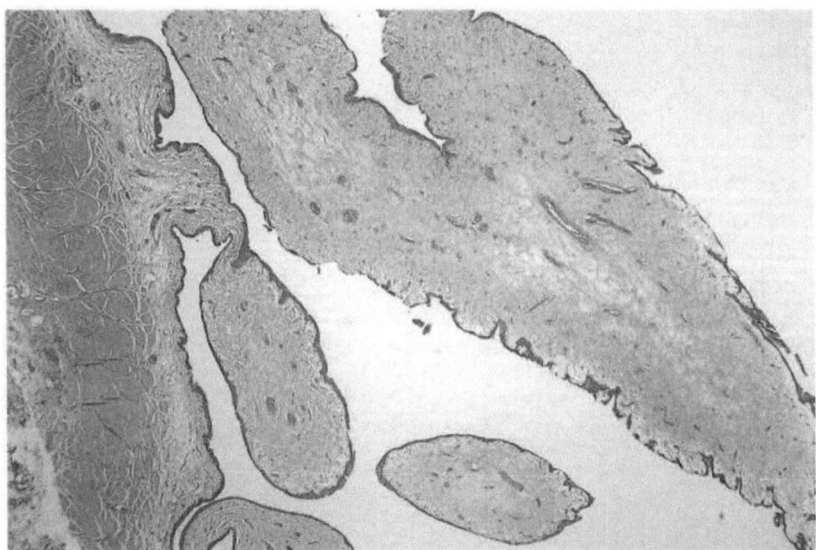

**Fig. 127.** *Fibroepithelial polyp*

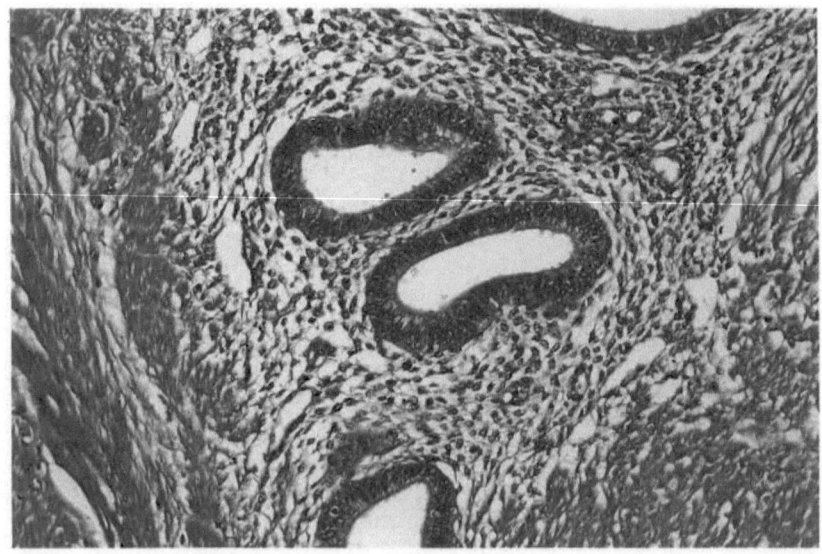

**Fig. 128.** *Endometriosis* in muscularis propria

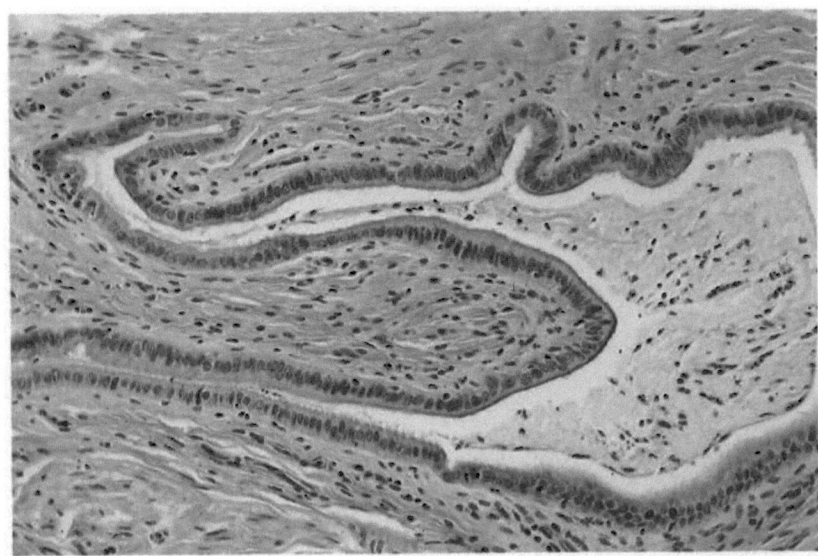

**Fig. 129.** *Endocervicosis*

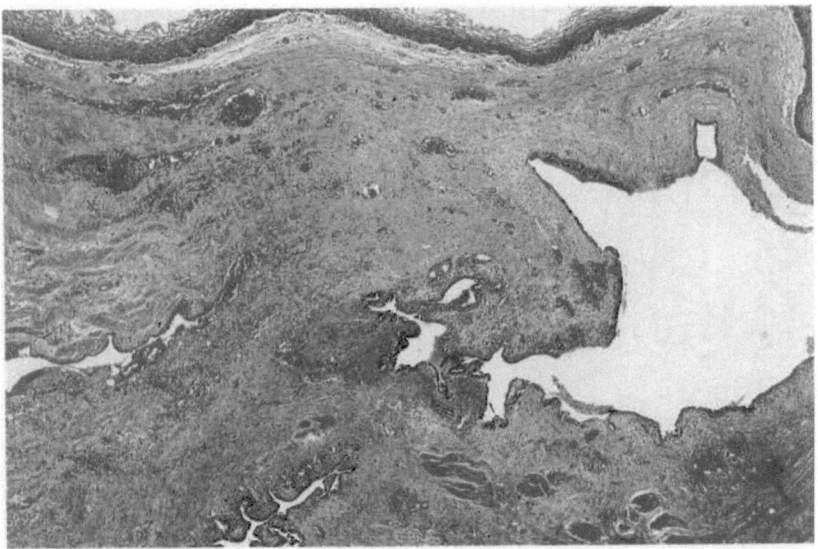

**Fig. 130.** *Trigonal cyst*

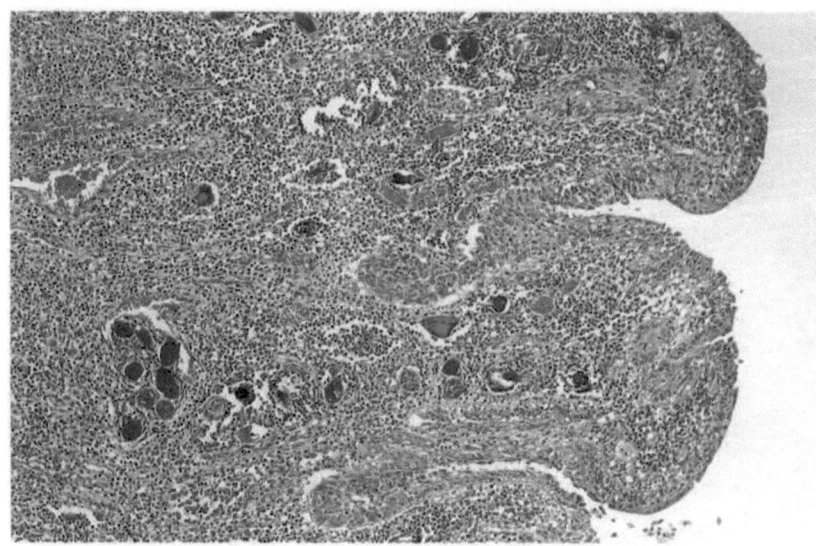

**Fig. 131.** *Schistosomiasis.* The inflammatory reaction has produced a polypoid tumour-like lesion

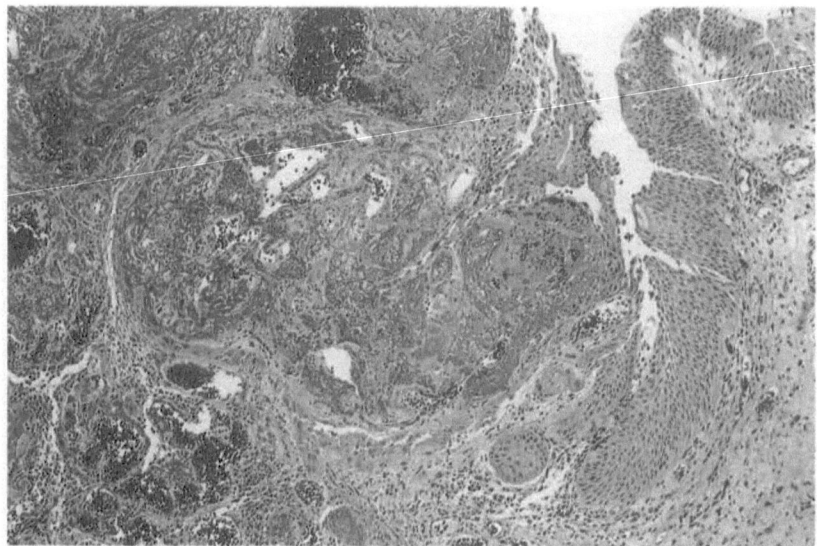

**Fig. 132.** *Radiation cystitis*

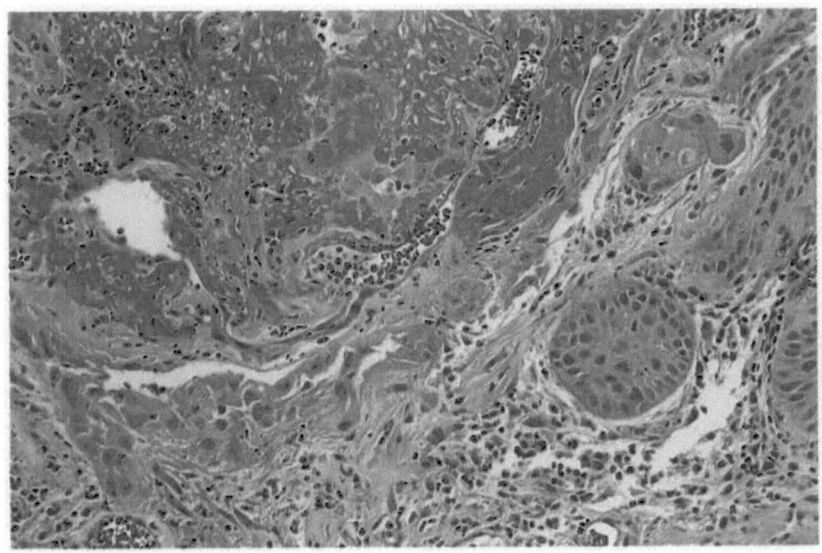

**Fig. 133.** *Radiation cystitis.* Higher magnification of Fig. 132

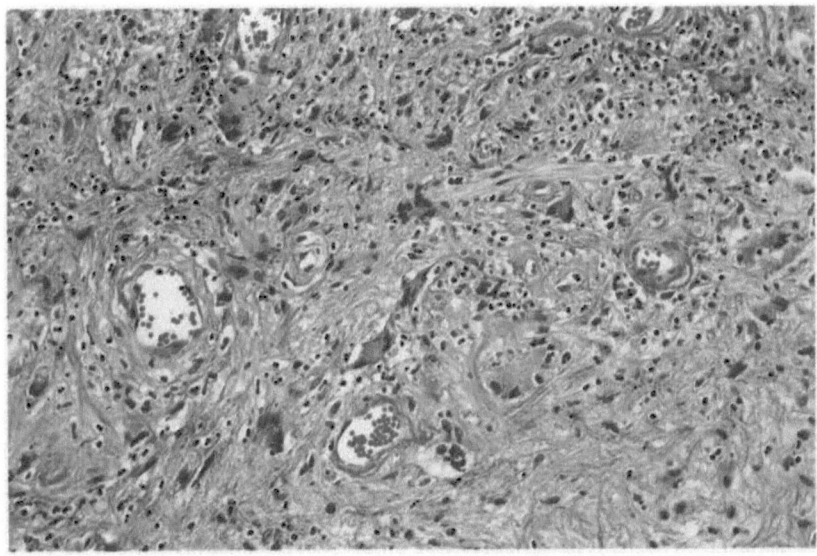

**Fig. 134.** *Giant cell cystitis.* This lesion is most often seen with radiation cystitis

# Subject Index